Effective Communication

A collection of articles
first published in The Professional Nurse
and here revised and updated

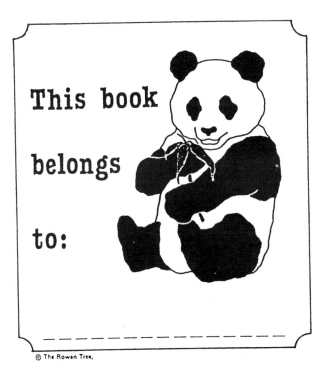

This book

belongs

to:

_____

© The Rowan Tree.

1990

Effective Communication
First published in 1990 by

Austen Cornish Publishers Limited
Austen Cornish House
Walham Grove
London SW6 1QW

ISBN 1 870065 14 X

Printed and bound in Great Britain by
Richard Clay Limited, Bungay, Suffolk

The Professional Developments Series

These five books provide you with a wealth of insight into all aspects of nursing practice. The series is essential reading for qualified, practising nurses who need to keep up with new developments, evaluate their clinical practice and develop and extend their clinical management and teaching skills. Up-to-date, and appropriately illustrated, The Professional Developments Series brings together the work of well over a hundred nurses.

Other titles in The Professional Developments Series:

The Ward Sister's Survival Guide
This book is essential reading and valuable reference for all nurses with direct clinical management responsibility.

The Staff Nurse's Survival Guide
Relevant to nurses working in all healthcare settings, this brings together chapters on a wide range of clinical and non-clinical issues in patient care, and includes a practical section on looking after *yourself* too.

Patient Education Plus
This book will help you to develop your teaching role with patients and clients, and covers a wide range of clinical topics. Each chapter includes a clearly written and illustrated handout which can be freely photocopied or adapted for use with your clients.

Practice Check!
How well do you communicate with colleagues and patients? How do you respond when difficult situations arise? You can explore your responses to all these – and more – by using this book. Each Practice Check presents brief descriptions of situations which may arise in practice, together with open-ended questions and discussion to enable you to explore the problems and establish your own solutions.

These books are available from the publishers:

Austen Cornish Publishers Limited
Austen Cornish House
Walham Grove
London SW6 1QW   Tel: 01-381 6301

Ask to be included on their mailing list!

Contents

Introduction

Effective communication is an essential requirement wherever there are people living or working together. It becomes even more important when people are faced with change and uncertainty, frightening or anxiety-provoking situations and with trauma. At least one of these situations is likely to be the case at some stage for most people who become ill, or who are suffering from a chronic condition. Nurses and other health professionals will face these difficult situations as they work with their patients and, as members of a complex and diverse team, they also have a considerable interest in effective communication with their colleagues.

This book is developed from articles which were first published in *The Professional Nurse* magazine. They have been updated and brought together in this single volume. The first section on **communication skills** reviews the essential components of good communication and its value in clinical practice. The separate sections on **counselling** and **loss and bereavement** look in more depth at those groups of communication skills which are particularly valuable to nurses in many healthcare settings. The **teamwork** section explores some of the issues in communication between colleagues in the healthcare team and the section on **personal freedom** takes a critical and challenging view of our prejudices and assumptions about other people, and the way which these may inhibit effective communication. Practice Check!, another book in the Professional Development Series, contains a considerable amount of material which is also useful for readers exploring issues in effective communication. Practice Check! presents many of the situations which arise in nursing practice in which there are no clear 'right answers' and the majority of these have their basis in problems of communication. Each Practice Check enables you to explore your own approach to situations requiring effective communication with elderly people, children, anxious people, those who are dying or in pain, and could be used alongside this book.

Elizabeth M. Horne,
Editorial Director, The Professional Nurse,
London, November 1989

Communication Skills

1

Empathy: the key to understanding

Philip Burnard, MSc, RGN, RMN, DipN, Cert Ed, RNT
Lecturer in Nursing, University of Wales College of Medicine, Heath Park, Cardiff

To fully understand another person seems a worthy aim in most aspects of nursing. The literature on the development of empathy as a vital prerequisite of skilled nursing is growing (Anthony and Carkhuff, 1976; Pluckhan, 1978). This chapter looks at practical methods of developing empathy, those which may be used by individuals working alone, or in pairs or groups – perhaps in training settings. This variety of approaches may be used as they stand, or adapted for use in basic nurse education or on counselling and other interpersonal skills training courses in continuing nurse education.

The problems and methods described here are relevant to both clinical and tutorial staff. The training guidelines can be used in both clinical and education settings.

True understanding

Empathy is the ability to see the world as another person sees it: to enter another's 'frame of reference'. We all view the world according to our own cultural background, educational experiences, belief and value systems and personal experiences. What happens to us as we grow up colours the way we perceive the world. To empathise is to attempt to set aside our *own* perception of things and attempt to think the way the other person thinks, or feel the way he feels. It is a very different quality or skill to sympathy. Sympathy involves 'feeling sorry' for the other person – or, perhaps, it involves our imagining how *we* would feel like if *we* were experiencing what is happening to him. With empathy, we try to image what it is like *being* the other person and experiencing things as he does. Sympathy is rarely as valuable a quality as empathy.

Empathy is the basis for truly understanding another person. It is the basis of any interpersonal relationship and has many implications for nursing. Until nurses can empathise with others they cannot attempt to understand what hospitalisation means to patients. Empathising can help nurses to appreciate other people's pain or distress, indeed most aspects of nursing can probably be aided by its development.

It does, of course, have its limits. In the end, it is impossible to *completely* enter someone else's frame of reference: to *exactly* experience the world as they do. It is important, though, that nurses try: if not, they will assume that other people's experience is similar to their own, and lose sight of the fact that other people live different lives, believe different things and feel different feelings. Nurses' attention should focus on understanding others: empathy can help to do this.

Individual development of empathy

The development of empathy is therefore important in all branches of nursing. Empathy training may be introduced into introductory blocks developed throughout training and continued into further education programmes. So how can individuals develop the ability to empathise?

The main method for individual development can become a way of life. It involves the ability to fully focus one's senses on the other person and to resist the temptation to rush to 'interpret' what the other person says or does. Thus the nurse must sit and fully observe the other person. She must listen to the patient, observe his nonverbal behaviour and register all this without any attempt at judging or categorising what he says or does.

This is different to 'normal' conversation, where one usually checks constantly to see whether or not what the other person says or does fits in with one's own belief or value system. Usually, too, one is rehearsing what one is about to say, and thus not fully attending to the other person. The method being described here suggests that it is valuable merely to sit and absorb all aspects of the other person while suspending judgement upon them. In doing so, one enters the other person's perceptual world, forgetting temporarily one's own viewpoint.

Clearing a space

This ability to fully focus on the other person is not easy. It is particularly difficult if the nurse is under pressure to think, or do, other things. When she is busy or distracted by her own problems, the ability to give her attention fully to the other person is reduced. With practice, however, it is possible to set aside her own pressures and problems in order to create the right conditions for true attention. Gendlin (1981) describes this well and calls it 'clearing a space'.

Briefly stated, 'clearing a space' involves an individual quietly reflecting upon the distractions that are going through her mind, and then finding ways of setting aside each of those distractions in turn until she is able to focus attention clearly on the other person. Some people find it useful to imagine each 'distraction' being packaged up in some way and temporarily being put to one side. This is not to say that this process somehow 'cures' the problems or distractions the aim, is merely to pull away from them for a while to give attention to others. Clearing a space and offering full attention in this way can be developed by a nurse working on her own.

Focusing attention Focusing attention fully on the other person involves a conscious decision. We have to decide that, for the next few minutes, we will give our time totally to the other person. This conscious element of the skill allows us to train ourselves. Because it is a conscious effort, we can *decide* to engage in it or not to engage in it, as the case may be. This process has been called 'conscious use of self' (Heron, 1977) and is listed as a skill in the 1982 Syllabus of Training for Psychiatric Nurses (ENB, 1982).

Training ourselves to give others our attention in this way can enhance our listening ability, make us more accurate as communicators and is the basic requirement for the development of empathy. If we are not truly concentrating on the other person, we cannot empathise with them.

Working in pairs

An elaboration of the self-training described above is empathy training in pairs. This method may be used as a training tool in a variety of nurse education settings.

The simplest two-way exercise involves two people, A and B, sitting opposite each other. A talks to B for five minutes while B listens and does not comment. After five minutes, the roles are reversed and B talks to A while A listens passively. The aim of this exercise is to develop the concentration. The exercise is *not* a conversation but an attempt at exploring, fully, the process of completely attending to another person. When both A and B have taken turns as talkers and listeners, they can discuss the process of the exercise. Pertinent questions here are: 'What was it like to really listen?' and 'What was it like to be listened to?'

An elaboration of this exercise involves A listening to B and then offering B a paraphrase of what she has just said. This is a difficult exercise – what we *hear* and what we *think* we hear are often two different things. Once A has accurately paraphrased B's talk (to B's satisfaction), the roles are again reversed.

Reflection A third exercise in empathy building for use in pairs uses the same format. A talks to B who uses only reflection as a response in the conversation. Reflection is a counselling intervention skill described by Egan (1982), Burnard (1985) and others and involves repeating the last few words of an utterance back to the talker. Alternatively, the response may be a brief paraphrase of what the person has just said. The following conversation demonstrates the use of reflection:

A: "When I first came into hospital, I felt completely alone and that nobody would come and see me."

B: "You thought that no one would come and see you..."

A: "Well, I knew my husband would, but I wasn't so sure about the rest of the family – particularly my older children."

B: "You weren't too sure about the family..."

A: "We've quite a large family and they mostly live a long way away..."

In this example, the use of reflection allows the nurse to try to enter the perceptual frame of the client without imposing other ideas and without adding anything to what the client says. So, in this exercise B responds to A by using only reflection and thus practises the process of developing empathy. One drawback to this exercise is that both A and B are 'in the know' about the use of reflection, and sometimes the exercise can feel rather contrived. It is worth saying, however, that if this contrivance is acknowledged, many people find that 'practising' in this way is a useful aid to developing the skill of reflection (and thus empathy development) in real life.

It is not suggested that reflection is the *only* method of response to a client's conversation, nor that it is the *only* method of displaying empathy. It is one among many further empathic interventions described in the counselling literature (Nelson-Jones, 1981).

Group method

There is also a method of training in empathy development that may be used by groups of about five to 15. Fewer than this can make the exercise too easy and thus insufficiently challenging: numbers greater than this can lead to the development of subgroups or 'groups within groups'. If larger groups are to attempt this exercise it is useful to break them up and run a number of smaller groups concurrently.

This exercise is one that Carl Rogers used in empathy development as part of his counselling skills training courses (Kirshenbaum, 1979). It involves running a group discussion on any topic with one 'ground rule': that once someone has spoken, the next person to speak must summarise the last contribution to the satisfaction of that person before she offers her own contribution. Thus the exercise is an elaboration of the one described earlier for use in pairs. It requires the group members to listen closely to each other. The facilitator running the group should ensure that the 'ground rule' is adhered to and that the summary made satisfies the person who last contributed.

It is useful to run such an exercise for a set period of time, say 45 minutes, and then hold a discussion for 30 minutes about what the experience was like. It is important that this discussion focuses on *what the experience was like* and does not become an extension of the topic discussed in the exercise. It is sometimes important, too, for the facilitator to point out that the ground rule need not apply to the discussion.

These practical exercises may each be used to enhance empathy. All three may be combined for use in nurse education. The individual focus is useful as an ongoing discipline for the nurse in training. The pairs exercises are valuable as introductory exercises in human relations training, and the group activity is useful as a means of developing empathy towards a number of people. It is particularly effective for nurses who, as part of their job, run groups of any sorts. Many other exercises are available and the reader is recommended to explore the literature (Canfield and Wells, 1976; Francis and Young, 1979).

Problems in empathy training

What are some of the problems that may arise in empathy training? The first is, perhaps, the reticence of some nurses to take part in these activities at all. It is important that any such participation is voluntary and, paradoxically, the more freedom people are given to 'sit out' on these exercises, the more readily they usually join in! It is important, then, that any abstentions are respected. It is also important that any empathy-building exercises used are clearly set up and that an accurate rationale for their use is offered to those taking part.

A second problem that sometimes arises is that people find the exercises artificial. This point has been dealt with to some degree already. It is important to acknowledge the criticism but, equally, it is important to acknowledge the *value* of this skills training. It may be analogous to learning how to give an injection: this is often taught using inanimate objects to represent the person, so the basic techniques are learned and can then be transferred to the 'real' situation. So it is with empathy training. The initial steps are 'tried out' in the educational setting: the basic skills learned can then be used in 'real life'.

It is important to note that skills training of this sort is *not* role play, but a form of direct experiential learning. Role play invites people to act out roles other than their real-life one. In skills training of the above sort, all participants remain 'themselves': they are *not* acting out a role.

A third potential problem is that of time. As with all forms of experiential learning, the activities described above (if they are done properly) take considerable time. It is particularly important that the follow-up discussions after the activities are lengthy. This is the time when new perceptions are being formed and new learning takes place. It is of little use to merely undertake the exercise without considerable reflection upon it afterwards. It is recommended that only *one* exercise is tackled in a session of at least two hours.

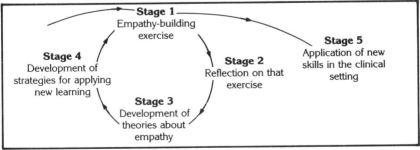

Figure 1. The experiential learning cycle.

Learning gained from empathy-building sessions can be incorporated readily into everyday nursing practice. Figure 1 outlines the experiential learning cycle (Burnard, 1985) which identifies the stages involved in learning through the exercises described here. In stage one, the exercise is undertaken by the individual, pair or group. In stage two, reflection upon that experience can lead to the third stage – that of developing theories about how empathy 'works'. In stage four, new strategies are designed so that the new learning may be applied, and in stage five, the nurse uses her new skills in the clinical situation.

A lifelong process

Empathy development is a lifelong process. It does not start, or finish with a selection of exercises. However, training does enable the issues of empathy to be addressed and enhances the nurse's natural empathic ability.

This natural ability is of prime importance. Skills training cannot give people sensitivity or respect for others, but, based as it is on the individual nurse's experience, it can do much to develop those qualities. One cannot leave the ability to empathise to chance, nor imagine that it will somehow develop throughout a course of training.

It is important that empathy training is not seen only as the concern of the nurse education unit. The training methods described here can be used by those working in the clinical setting – whether ward- or community-based. For example, it is possible for the exercises described here to be used as the basis of a series of clinical seminars. In this way, the learning gained has direct application. There need be no gap between 'theory' and practice. The skills are both *learned* and *used* in the clinical setting. The nurse needs empathy to fire the relationship between her and the patient, so it would seem valuable to learn the art and skill of empathising as close to the patient as possible.

References

Anthony, W.C. and Carkhuff, R.R. (1976) The Art of Health Care: A Handbook of Psychological First Aid Skills. Human Resource Development Press, Massachusetts.

Burnard, P. (1985) Learning Human Skills: A Guide for Nurses. Heinemann, London.

Canfield J. and Wells, H.C. (1976) 100 Ways to Enhance Self-Concept in the Classroom. Prentice-Hall, New Jersey.

Egan, G. (1982) The Skilled Helper (2nd edn). Brooks/Cole, Monterery.

ENB (1982) Syllabus of Training: Professional Register: Part 3 (Registered Mental Nurse). ENB, London.

Francis, D. and Young, D. (1979) Improving Work Groups: A Practical Manual for Team Building. University Associates, San Diego, California.

Gendlin, E. (1981) Focussing, Basic Books, New York.

Heron J. (1977) Behaviour Analysis in Education and Training: Human Potential Research Project. University of Surrey, Guildford.

Kirschenbaum, H. (1979) On Becoming Carl Rogers. Dell, New York.

Le Shan, L. (1974) How to Meditate. Turnstone Press, Wellingborough.

Nelson-Jones, R. (1981) The Theory and Practice of Counselling Psychology. Holt, Rinehart and Winston, London.

Pluckhan, M.L. (1978) Human Communication: The Matrix of Nursing. McGraw Hill, New York.

2

Developing skills as a group facilitator

Philip Burnard, MSc RGN RMN DipN Cert Ed RNT
Lecturer in Nursing, School of Nursing Studies, University of Wales College of Medicine, Cardiff

Nurses are frequently called upon to run groups of various sorts. In general hospitals they may organise and run case conferences, teaching sessions and quality circles, and in psychiatric and mental handicap hospitals they may be active participants in group therapy as well as being engaged in educational activities of various sorts. Group facilitation calls for the exercise of particular and specific skills. As well as needing a thorough knowledge of group processes and dynamics, the nurse is required to use a variety of verbal interventions to keep the group going.

This chapter identifies three sets of facilitator behaviour that will enable the nurse to choose the appropriate type of verbal intervention for the particular group at a particular moment. The sets are based on the behaviour analyses of John Heron (1977) and Rackham and Morgan (1977). Group dynamics, group activities or procedure are not discussed. The aim is to offer a practical framework that the nurse may use while conducting groups of various sorts. Some ideas are offered of the types of group interventions available which can be developed further by the group facilitation training offered by many colleges and university departments. Such training is increasingly becoming part of basic and continuing nurse education.

Framework

The framework offers three groups of possible verbal interventions focusing on three different aspects of time: recent past, present and future. The headings of those groups are:
- clarifying recent talk;
- developing current talk;
- initiating further talk.

By an appropriate mix of the three types of intervention, the nurse can facilitate a group discussion that is continuous, dynamic and lively — not that such interventions can be learned by rote. The particular words chosen are dependent upon a variety of things, including, at least: the context, the nurse's own background and personality and the particular needs of the group at the time. The headings and the examples that follow are, therefore, guidelines to verbal behaviour — they suggest methods of making interventions: they are not examples of specific verbal statements. Each of the three groups will now be broken down into examples of methods.

Clarifying recent talk

Here, the nurse uses interventions to enable the group to be clear about what is and what is not under discussion. Some of the methods that may be used to clarify are:

Summary   Offering a summing up of the group discussion so far, and a clear and accurate statement of the main threads and issues of the preceding talk.

Inter-relate   Indicating how various points under discussion link together to form a cohesive whole.

Disagree   Suggesting a reasoned alternative to what has gone before as a means of clarifying and leading on to further discussion.

These are three methods the nurse may use to clarify recent talk within the group. Such interventions may be used periodically throughout the group meeting or whenever there seems to be misunderstanding.

Developing current talk

Interventions are used to further draw out group members on the subject under discussion. They are similar in nature to the sorts of interventions used in non-directive or client centred counselling. Some of the methods the nurse may use here are:

Reflection   Repeating the last few words said by a group member to enable that person to further develop what they have said. Alternatively, the nurse may paraphrase the last few statements to similar effect. This is sometimes known as 'echoing' or 'mirroring'.

Checking for understanding   Rephrasing something a group member has said and checking whether or not that restatement represents a clearer version of what was meant. Alternatively, the nurse asks the direct question: ''are you saying that . . .?''

Support   Agreeing with or encouraging the statement made by a group member in order to promote further discussion.

These are basic methods that may be used throughout a group meeting. They are encouraging and promote the development of group cohesion.

Initiate further talk

Interventions are used to encourage the group to move on and to develop further. Some of the methods that may be used here are:

Propose   Suggesting a new direction for a new topic for consideration by the group. The group is then free to adopt or reject the proposal as it chooses. Alternatively, the nurse may wish to consult the group first about a plan of action and then make a proposal arising out of that consultation: a 'consult, then propose' format.

Question A variety of open questions are posed to encourage movement within the group. Generally speaking, questions that begin with 'why' are best avoided. 'Why' questions tend to sound interrogative; they can sound moralistic and they can lead to sterile theoretical discussion that only impede group development.

Disclose As facilitator, the nurse offers the group personal thoughts, feelings or experiences. Disclosure begets disclosure. The nurse who reveals something about herself sets an example to the group of openness which may encourage further disclosure on the part of group members.

These methods may be used to encourage the group to develop, to stretch itself and to move into new areas. They need to be timed accurately paying regard to the atmosphere at the time. If they are used too often or too quickly they may not be well received. On the other hand, if they are used deftly, they can ensure that the group continues to develop.

Conscious use of self

Other group interventions that do not easily fit within the three groups above may be identified. The nurse may, for instance, bring in a group member who contributes little by asking for their thoughts or feelings on a particular matter. On the other hand, the nurse may gently shut out the over-talkative member who may tend to lionise the group. Both these interventions need to be used with tact and sensitivity.

Sometimes the nurse will offer specific information. Again, 'information giving' needs to be well timed. We have all experienced facilitators, teachers and chairpeople who offer too much information. Group facilitation should be concerned more with *sharing* ideas than with dispensing information.

Interventions so far described may be practised through conscious use within a particular group. In other words the nurse monitors herself and chooses only to use these sorts of interventions. Such self monitoring takes concentration and practice. It is a form of what Heron (1977) calls 'conscious use of self' and such use of self is now defined as a skill in the psychiatric nursing student's syllabus of training (ENB, 1982).

Such conscious use of self is an important aspect of group facilitation. It suggests that the group facilitator pays close attention to what is said and done while the group is running. Thus, group facilitation becomes a task of greater precision — little is left to chance. Group facilitation is, after all, a skilled task — it is not something that needs to be regarded as 'coming naturally to some and not to others'. We would not say this of other nursing skills, nor need we say it of the interpersonal aspects of nursing.

Theoretical assumptions

Other aspects of group facilitation that may be considered by the nurse include: coping with silences; dealing with decision making; opening and closing groups; dealing with 'difficult' members and so forth. Again, such aspects of group work can be learned through training courses and through the experience of working with groups.

Anyone who runs a group does so from a particular theoretical position — they have a theory about how people act in groups. This may be clearly thought out or it may be something of which the nurse is only dimly aware. It pays considerable dividends to explore these underlying theoretical assumptions before setting out to organise and run a group. One method is to write down in note form a series of assumptions, followed by an attempt to justify those assumptions. The process of doing this can help to clarify values, beliefs and assumptions about people in groups, some of which will have been adopted through nurse training. Psychiatric nurses, for instance, will probably tend to hold a number of assumptions about 'group psychology' based within one or more of the three broad categories: behavioural, psychodynamic or humanistic. It is worth clarifying these before group work is undertaken.

Awareness and skill

The framework offered here may be used as a typography of verbal behaviours for use in research. It can be used in quantitative research for categorising types of observed behaviour in group activities, and it also has applications in more qualitative work to explore group processes in participant-observer studies.

Nurses working with groups need a sound theoretical basis for the work, a thorough grounding in practical facilitation skills and an awareness of research into groups. After experience as group facilitators, they may then add to the body of knowledge by conducting their own research. In this way, nurse facilitation can develop both as a dynamic science and as an art.

Example of the group at work

The group is a small number of student nurses in the nurse education centre. The facilitator is a newly qualified nurse who is using a facilitative approach to discussing the concept of counselling.

As the session unfolds Jane continues to use facilitative interventions only and thus allows the group to explore *their own* thoughts and feelings without offering direct suggestions or prescriptions of her own. Notice, too, that Jane's *own* disclosure prompted the disclosure of others.

This, then, is one application of the framework — to *consciously* use interventions from the three categories. After a while the categories are internalised and the need to make such conscious decisions becomes less important. By this time, the facilitative style has become the person's natural style.

Group Discussion	Example from the framework
Jane (tutor) "Do you think nurses *should* be trained as counsellors?	Initiating further talk (question).
Samantha (student) "No, not really!"	
Jane "You don't feel they should?"	Developing current talk (reflection)
Samantha "It should be left to people trained as counsellors . . ."	
Peter (student) "But we are trained as counsellors."	
Samantha "Not enough, though . . . . not to do it properly . . ."	
Jane "So . . . one of you thinks nurses should counsel and you're not so sure.	Clarifying recent talk (summary)
Jane "What are other people's views?	Initiating further talk (question)
Silence	
Jane "I feel slightly uncomfortable . . . I'd hoped that you'd all have something to say . . ."	Initiating further talk (self-disclosure)
Ruth (student): "I think that counselling is important as long as we all know what we are doing . . . you know . . . properly trained"	
Samantha: "Do you know all about it then?	
Ruth "No, but I'm learning.	
Peter to Samantha: "You're very aggressive today! Why are you so negative?"	
Samantha: "I just think we've got to be clear, that's all . . . I didn't mean to sound negative . . . I only hope we get more practical work on counselling.	

Bibliography

Berger, G. and Berger, P. (1972) Group Training Techniques. Gower, Aldershot.
This offers an overview of group training processes and practical activities for group skills development.

Bion, W. (1961) Experiences in Groups. Tavistock, London.
A classic work on the psychodynamic view of group development.

Burnard, P. (1985) Learning Human Skills: A Guide for Nurses. Heinemann, London.
A practical handbook containing the theory of self-awareness and experiential learning. It also offers a range of exercises for counselling and group facilitation skills development.

Cartwright, D. and Zander, A. (1968) Group Dynamics: Research and Theory. 3rd Edition. Tavistock, London.
A comprehensive volume of almost all aspects of group dynamics and processes.

Francis, D. and Young, D. (1979) Improving Work Groups: A Practical Manual for Team Building. University Associates, California.
A useful compendium of activities for developing group skills.

Heron, J. (1977) Dimensions of Facilitator Style: Human Potential Research Project. University of Surrey, Guildford. Contains a presentation of six dimensions of group facilitation.
A useful guide to both the theory and the practice of group facilitation.

Schulman, E.D. (1982) Intervention in Human Services: A Guide to Skills and Knowledge. 3rd Edition. C.V. Mosby, Toronto.
A comprehensive account of various approaches to interpersonal skills training.

Smith, P.B. (1980) Group Process and Personal Changes. Harper and Row, London.
A very thorough review of the literature on groups and group dynamics. Not always easy reading but very useful!

References

ENB (1982) Syllabus of training: Part 3 Registered Mental Nurse.

Heron, J. (1977) Behaviour Analysis in Education and Training: Human Potential Research Project. University of Surrey, Guildford.

Rackham, R. and Morgan, J. (1977) Behaviour Analysis in Training. McGraw Hill, London.

3
Encouraging compliance

Ruth E. Smith, BSc, RGN, RMN, DNCert
Support Worker in Rehabilitation, Lothian Regional Council, Department of Social Work.

Jill Birrell, MA(Hons), MSc, AFBPsS, C.Psychol,
Clinical Psychologist, Royal Edinburgh Hospital

'Non-compliance is not restricted to medicine. Not every bit of advice given by solicitors, architects, business consultants and other professionals is followed by those who have sought their services. Clients exercise their judgement, as is their right, when presented with professional advice even though they may not have the experience claimed by their advisers . . . clients' failure to follow advice may have serious consequences, yet these professions tend to see this independence as part of a client's rights and if they study non-compliance at all, do not do so in terms of client deficiency but in terms of necessary improvement in the services they offer.' (Thompson, 1984).

Compliance is generally used to refer to adherence or co-operation — doing as the health professional says concerning health matters. Taking medicine when one is supposed to, going on a prescribed diet or stopping smoking when advised are all examples of compliance. Non-compliance, may cause a breakdown in a treatment programme. It may put an individual at risk of a more serious illness or prolong the current difficulty.

Studies published

An early study by Stockwell (1972) describes the views of nurses in the inpatient setting where patients are described as 'popular' or 'unpopular'. 'Popular' patients are passive in interactions with staff, unquestioning and undemanding. Patients who question their treatment and express views about the nursing care they receive are regarded as 'unpopular'. Perhaps unpopularity and non-compliance have similarities?

Compared with inpatient settings, hospital outpatient clinics and general practice consultations have far greater difficulties regarding compliance – they have a less captive audience. Non-compliance can take many forms, among them failure to turn up for an appointment, failure to file prescriptions, discontinuing medication early, failure to make recommended changes in daily routine and missing follow-up appointments. Studies of a wide variety of illnesses, including coronary heart disease, hypertension, glaucoma and diabetes, have indicated that only 40 to 70 per cent of patients comply fully with physicians' prescriptions and advice. It is also worth noting that problems of non-compliance are often aggravated in elderly people who have no family support to ensure they follow instructions correctly. Macdonald et al (1977) found that twelve weeks after discharge from hospital, half of the elderly people studied were taking less than 50 per cent of their tablets while a further 25 per cent were seriously overdosing themselves. Less than 25 per cent were still taking medicine as prescribed. Clearly consultations often fail to convince patients of the wisdom of the proposed treatment.

Peck (1978) noted that a large number of studies have endeavoured to find an association between compliance and demographic variables such as sex, educational level, age, race, income and religion. If an association is present at all, it is very low. Studies have also been conducted on disease variables and it has been found that the diagnosis, severity of illness, duration of illness, previous hospitalisation and degree of illness or disability also have little or no association with compliance. The only reasonably consistent finding seems to be that psychiatric patients tend to be less compliant than patients with a physical illness.

Most important factors in determining the degree of compliance are more subjective than objective. Patients' satisfaction with contacts with health professionals and beliefs about illness are important. Rosenstock (1966) and Becker (1974) present the Health Belief Model (Table 1).

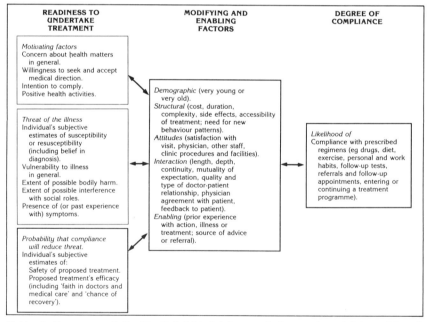

Table 1. Summary of Health Belief Model for predicting and explaining sick role behaviour, adapted from Becker, M.H.: The health belief model and sick-role behaviour reproduced with kind permission of the Society for Public Health Education, Inc.

Clearly patients' readiness to act is paramount. Action comes from their perception of the severity of the disease or possible progression and their perceived susceptibility to illness. If a patient does not believe that an illness is serious or does not believe he or she is likely to become ill, the readiness to act is low, whereas if the patient believes the illness is severe and there is a high chance of him or her contracting it, readiness to act is high. Important too are patients' considerations of the costs and benefits of compliance. They must believe that treatment will be effective.

Increasing compliance

Patients must understand and remember advice if they are to pay attention to it. Compliance is likely to be higher if the doctor or other health professional has a warm and friendly manner, heeds the patient's need for information, talks about non-medical topics and tests out and corrects any misunderstandings the patient may have. Written information seems effective in improving compliance in the short term. Categorisation of material into blocks has also proved useful. For example, saying "I am going to tell you what you must do to help yourself, what treatment you will receive, what tests need to be done" and suchlike, leads to greater recall of information. Also, the more specific the information given, the more compliance will be achieved. Telling a patient to lose half a stone is more effective than simply saying that he or she must lose weight. Supervision by a health worker can effectively increase compliance, as the act of reporting regularly to someone is reinforcing to the patient. When that constant supervision is removed, however, compliance returns to its lower initial rates. Finally, attempts to improve the communication skills of health care workers by further teaching and discussion have also shown promise. Research must continue to look for ways of removing barriers that prevent patients working well with health professionals and as Thompson (1974) states "a fuller understanding of attitude change required if the generally poor record of medical advisers is to be improved".

Bibliography
Fitzpatrick, R. et al. (1984) The Experience of Illness. Tavistock Publications, London and New York.
    The most comprehensive discussion of the literature to date. The book covers most areas of patients' experiences of illness.
Gatchel, R.J. and Baum, A. (1983) An Introduction to Health Psychology. Addison Wesley Publishing Company, London.
    Easier reading than Fitzpatrick et al – covers patients' experiences of illness but with less research data. Chapter seven is a precise summary of the main points.
Rachman, S.J. and Phillips, C. (1978) Psychology and Medicine. Penguin Publications, London.
    Chapter three is a short introductory text.

References
Becker, M.H. (1974) The health belief model and sick role behaviour. *Health Education Mongraph*, **2**, 409-419.

MacDonald, E.T., MacDonald, J.B. and Phoenix, M. (1977) Improving drug compliance after hospital discharge. *British Medical Journal* **2,** 618-621.

Peck, D. (1987) Communication and compliance. *Bulletin of the British Psychological Society,* **32,** 348-352.

Rosenstock. I.M. (1966) Why people use health services. *Millbank Memorial Fund Quarterly,* 94-127.

Stockwell, F. (1972) The unpopular patient. Royal College of Psychiatrists, Series 1, No. 2.

Thompson, J. (1984) Compliance. In Fitzpatrick, R., Hinton, J., Newman, S., Scambler, G. and Thompson, J. (Eds) (1984) The Experience of Illness.Tavistock Publications, London and New York.

The authors are aware that there are no references listed from nursing journals. There appears to be a lack of significant and relevant reports in this area of nursing.

4
Confidentiality

Elizabeth M. Horne, MA
Editorial Director, The Professional Nurse

The Code of Professional Conduct (UKCC, 1984) states that: registered nurses, midwives and health visitors shall: "Respect confidential information obtained in the course of professional practice and refrain from disclosing such information without the consent of the patient/client, or a person entitled to act on his/her behalf, except where disclosure is required by law or by the order of a court, or is necessary in the public interest."

Conflicts in practice
Isolated from practice, this statement may seem reasonable, but practitioners are daily faced with decisions based on the application of these principles in situations which may contain inherent conflicts of interest. They need confident, working definitions of the elements involved, and to establish clear priorities between the expectations of their patients and those of a wider public. Not so easy when, for example, a sister in a psychiatric day hospital finds a patient in possession of large quantities of controlled drugs that he cannot have obtained legally, or an occupational health nurse is asked by her manager for information about an employee. These examples are cited by the UKCC in a new advisory paper on confidentiality (UKCC, 1987), which suggests that the most difficult problem for practitioners is identifying and establishing the boundary between clients' expectations that information will not be disclosed, and the expectations of the public that they will not be unreasonably put at risk.

Confidentiality is important for effective communication
The knowledge that confidentiality will be respected is important for effective communication. There is much information people would not discuss with anyone unless they knew the recipient was completely trustworthy in their offer of confidentiality. Without this trust they may choose to keep quiet, which could affect their health.

Standards of confidentiality should be made clear to clients
It is not practicable to obtain clients' consent every time information needs to be shared with other health professionals, so it should be made known to all clients what standards of confidentiality are maintained.

The practitioner who holds the information must ensure, as far as possible, that it is imparted in strict professional confidence and for a specific purpose serving interests of the client. An individual practitioner is responsible for deciding when it is necessary to obtain the explicit consent of a patient or client.

Practitioners must be familiar with how record systems are used, who has access to them and what are the risks to confidentiality associated with their use. Where students, or those involved in research, require access to records, the same principles of confidentiality apply, and the patient's consent must be sought where appropriate, and the use of the records closely supervised.

Breaches of confidentiality

The principle of confidentiality must be the rule, and breaches of it exceptional; the practitioner must be sure that the best interests of theclient, or thoseof confidential information. The interests of the community may, occasionally, take precedence over those of an individual.

The withholding or disclosing of confidential information may have serious consequences, and the practitioner's decision can be extremely difficult. However, the responsibility cannot be delegated. The individual practitioner must make the decision, and must be able to justify it. It may be helpful to make a written note of the decision and reasons for it on the file for future reference. Situations of this nature can be very stressful, and if other practitioners are aware of them, it may be helpful to discuss the problems. However it is still the responsibility of the individual practitioner, and he or she must ultimately make their own decision.

The UKCC Advisory Paper on Confidentiality is available from: UKCC, 23 Portland Place, London W1N 3AF (send a S.A.E.). It discusses the responsibility of individual practitioners for confidentiality, and the everyday implications for practice, the ownership and care of information, and some of the issues which arise when confidentiality is deliberately breached.

References

United Kingdom Central Council for Nursing, Midwifery and Health Visiting, (1984). Code of Professional Conduct for the Nurse, Midwife and Health Visitor. Second Edition. UKCC, London.

United Kingdom Central Council for Nursing, Midwifery and Health Visiting, (1987). Confidentiality: A UKCC Advisory Paper, UKCC, London.

5

What children think about hospitals and illness

Christine Eiser, BSc (Hons), PhD
Research Fellow, Department of Psychology, Washington Singer Laboratories, University of Exeter

Despite the enormous improvements made in caring for sick and hospitalised children since the publication of the Platt report (1959), admission to hospital is still a traumatic event. It is particularly traumatic for young children, who are much less well-informed than adults about ward procedures and treatments. Preschool children in particular may hold quite unpredictable views about what happens in hospitals. Redpath and Rogers (1984) found that some children believed that you went to hospital healthy and became ill while there. This and other research (Eiser and Patterson, 1984) has shown that young children may think that people in hospital always die, or that admission to hospital lasts for years, rather than days or weeks.

Less dramatically, but just as important in terms of how children perceive hospitals, is their confusion about the role of medical staff. In particular, Brewster (1982) showed that young children believed that doctors and nurses deliberately set out to hurt them, and this view was held even more strongly by children with a history of admissions compared with those with only brief experiences.

Punishment

Children differ greatly from adults in their understanding about the cause of illness, its treatment and prevention. There is some evidence that children's thoughts about illness change as they develop. Below seven years of age they may think that illness is a punishment for bad behaviour, or some magical rite.

They commonly think that all illnesses are contagious, and this may lead them to be suspicious of other children in the ward, fearing that they may 'catch' other illnesses (Bibace and Walsh, 1980). They do not understand how treatment can make them better, understandably — why should oral medication or an injection in the arm make a leg feel better?

Explanation of illness to children under seven must also take account of the fact that they have very limited understanding of their bodies (Crider, 1981; Eiser and Patterson, 1983) — they may be aware only that they have a heart, brain, blood and bones inside them. Awareness of their function is also very simple — the heart is for loving and the brain for 'doing sums'.

Misconceptions

Children between seven and 11 years become slightly more sophisticated, though their views are still by no means adult. Illness is caused by contact with 'germs', and there is still the belief that illness is generally spread by contact with others. They do not correctly infer the reasons for treatment. Beuf (1979) found that it was often assumed that a return to a normal diet was a sign of relapse, rather than improvement. By 11 years of age, children know they have a stomach and lungs. The stomach is 'for storing food' and children may not reliably be aware that food is converted to blood and waste. Commonly, they may think they have only one lung, and that they breathe through the mouth.

Increasing sophistication and adult-like concepts emerge from 11 years of age. In particular, children become aware that illness can be aggravated by psychological factors, and that stress or anxiety can influence the course of a disease. They become aware of the connections within the body — that there are digestive, respiratory or circulatory systems for example. Of particular importance, they realise that treatment sometimes makes them feel worse rather than better, and that it may be necessary to endure short-term discomfort in the hope of longer-term cure.

Effect of experience

This approach to understanding how children think about illness should be seen as an approximate guide. Their beliefs are likely to be affected by individual experiences — some children with chronic diseases, for example, can become relatively mature in their understanding, especially of their own disease. Others, particularly young chronically ill patients, may see only that their illness results in parental anxiety. This, and the fact that doctors and parents tend to keep young patients uninformed about their illness to avoid causing them stress, may mean that they remain less sophisticated in their reasoning than healthy children who have little experience of hospitals (Eiser et al, 1984).

In answering paediatric patients' questions, it is important to be aware of the limitations of their knowledge, and that answers may be interpreted very differently from how they were intended. Many medical terms are easily misinterpreted by children, for example, a diagnosis of diabetes may be taken to mean that a child will 'die of betes'; a diagnosis of oedema that 'there is a demon in my belly' (Perrin and Gerrity, 1981). It is also helpful to realise that many young patients believe that all illnesses are contagious, since this is likely to influence their behaviour on the ward.

How else may the stress of hospitalisation be reduced for young children? Undoubtedly it is important that they have some idea as to what to expect on a hospital ward. Generally, attempts to prepare children before admission have been successful in reducing anxiety and/or improving ward behaviour. Many American hospitals provide preparation for children being admitted for routine surgery (Azarnoff and Woody, 1981). The most common methods involve the use of films or videos (Melamed and Seigel, 1975), home visits by nurses (Ferguson, 1979), play therapy (Cassell and Paul, 1967), or pre-admission tours (McGarvey, 1983). Unfortunately, most of this preparation is aimed at the child being admitted for routine surgery and there is little in the way of preparation offered to chronically sick children. It is easy to forget that however minor and routine the procedures may appear to staff, they are potentially very frightening for children. Clearly, it is impossible to provide preparation for children admitted following traumatic injury, so there has been a move to provide children in the general community with information, so that they have some idea about what to expect should they require admission to hospital (McGarvey, 1983). Tours of hospitals appear to be enjoyed by young children, though it is not known if they result in less trauma for those who are later admitted.

Nurses can do a lot to reduce the stress of a child's hospital admission. Play and educational facilities which provide a continuity between home and hospital life are important. In recognising that children have different concerns from adults and by being aware that they are ill-informed about hospital and treatment, the nurse may be better able to answer a child's questions appropriately.

Children are given very little information about their illnesses directly by medical staff (Pantell et al, 1982), and may have to glean knowledge from eavesdropping adult conversation. This inevitably leads to misunderstanding. It is important for all health care professionals to appreciate the trauma hospital admission can cause to children and to ensure that they minimise its effect as much as possible.

References

Azarnoff, P. and Woody, P. (1981) Preparation of children for hospitalisation in acute care hospitals in the United States. *Pediatrics*, **68**, 361-8.

Beuf, A.H. (1979) Biting off the bracelet: a study of children in hospital. University of Pennsylvania Press, Philadelphia.

Bibace, R. and Walsh, M.E. (1980) Development of children's concepts of illness. *Pediatrics*, **66**, 913-17.

Brewster, A.B. (1982) Chronically ill hospitalised cheldren's concepts of their illness. *Pediatrics*, **69**, 355-362.

Cassell, S. and Paul, M. (1967) The role of puppet therapy on the emotional responses of children hospitalised for cardiac catheterisation. *Pediatrics*, **71**, 233-39.

Crider, C. (1981) Children's concepts of the body interior. In R. Bibace and M.E. Walsh (Eds.) Children's conceptions of health, illness and bodily functions. Jossey-Bass, San Francisco.

Eiser, C. and Patterson, D. (1983) "Slugs and snails and puppy-dog tails": children's ideas about the insides of their bodies. *Child: Care, Health and Development*, **9**, 233-40.

Eiser, C. and Patterson, D. (1984) Children's perceptions of hospital: a preliminary study. *International Journal of Nursing Studies*, **21**, 45-50.

Eiser, C., Patterson, D. and Tripp, J.H. (1984) Illness experience and children's conceptualisation of health and illness. *Child: Care, Health and Development*, **10**, 157-62.

Ferguson, B.F. (1979) Preparing young children for hospitalisation: a comparison of two methods. *Pediatrics*, **65**, 656-64.

McGarvey, M.E. (1983) Preschool hospital tours. *Children's Health Care,* 11, 12-24.

Melamed, B.C. and Siegel, L.J. (1975) Reduction of anxiety in children facing hospitalisation and surgery by use of filmed modelling. *Journal of Consulting and Clinical Psychology,* 43, 511-21.

Pantell, R.H., Stewart, T.J., Dias, J.K., Wells, P. and Ross, A.W. (1982) Physician communication with children and parents. *Pediatrics,* 70, 396-402.

Perrin, E.C. and Gerrity, P.S. (1981) There's a demon in your belly. Children's understanding of illness. *Pediatrics,* 67, 841-49.

Platt Committee, Great Britain (1959) The Welfare of Children in Hospitals. Her Majesty's Stationary Office, London.

Redpath, C. and Rogers, C.S. (1984) Healthy young children's concepts of hospitals, medical personnel, operations and illness. *Journal of Pediatric Psychology,* 9, 29-40.

6

Preparing children for hospital

Christine Eiser, BSc, PhD,
Research Fellow, Department of Psychology, University of Exeter

Lesley Hanson, BA, RSCN, HVCert,
School Nursing Sister, Exeter Health Authority

Hospital admission can be a frightening experience for children, particularly those who experience traumatic injury or sudden onset of chronic disease. To prepare them for the possibility of admission, it has been advocated that school-based education programmes be implemented (Elkins and Roberts, 1983; Peterson and Ridley-Johnson, 1983). This approach may also benefit children who are generally anxious about more routine visits to a doctor or dentist (Roberts et al, 1981).

One common approach to school-based intervention is the organised hospital tour. McGarvey (1983) reports that a programme for preschoolers, in which they were encouraged to "see, feel and experience" what happens in hospitals, was well received by children, teachers and parents. Three children who were subsequently hospitalised as emergency admissions were reported to adjust well.

An alternative technique involves setting up a 'play hospital' in school, and encouraging children to participate in both structured or free play situations (Brett, 1983). Elkins and Roberts (1984) set up a play hospital and used hospital volunteers dressed up as medical personnel to explain the equipment and procedures. The 25 children who took part in this activity subsequently reported fewer medical fears and were more knowledgeable about medical events than a control group of children.

Setting up a play hospital

This chapter is concerned with our own experiences in setting up a play hospital in primary schools, and describing the children's responses. The purpose of the study was twofold: to increase children's hospital related knowledge, and reduce anxiety and fear. Since some of the children were quite young, we did not feel verbally based assessments, such as interviews or questionnaires, were appropriate as the main techniques for evaluation. Instead, we focused on qualitative changes in the nature of children's play. Groups of three children were videotaped playing with the equipment on two separate occasions, four weeks apart. During the intervening period, children were given the opportunity to handle and play with the equipment under the guidance of a school nurse and mother helpers. We hoped that, as a result of experience with the equipment and a range of educational activities, we would be able to identify changes in play, reflecting improved knowledge and attitudes towards hospitals and medical personnel.

Method

Subjects   The children all attended a small first school (catering for five- to eight-year-olds) in a rural Devon town. There is little local industry, and unemployment is relatively high. The school, like most others in the district, caters for children predominantly from working and lower middle-class homes. None of the children suffered from any chronic condition, or had personal experience of hospital other than as an outpatient. Subjects were drawn from the reception class (five to 5½ years) and the third and fourth year (seven to eight years). They were collected from the classroom in groups of three (normally same-sex triads), selected by the teacher. Selection was random, rather than in terms of friendship patterns or ability levels. In all, 14 triads of five-year-olds and eight triads of eight-year-olds took part in the study.

Apparatus   A miniature hospital was set up in an empty classroom in the school. It was divided into four areas.

- The **reception** area consisted of a table and two chairs opposite each other. On the table was a telephone, notepad and pencil. There was also a display rack containing a selection of health education leaflets.
- The **hospital ward** consisted of two beds made with blankets, and a baby's cot, complete with doll. There was a food table on one of the beds, and a 'drip' hanging at the side. On a small table nearby were several pairs of rubber gloves, cotton facemasks and head covers (of the type used in surgery). On a series of open shelves was an array of medical equipment, including a stethoscope, syringe, tweezers, respiratory mask and nursing bowls.
- In the **X-ray** area was a hard table covered with a sheet. Above the table was a pretend light that could be swung through a semicircle, and two X-rays were hung on the wall.
- In the **surgery** areas, another hard table was covered by a sheet. There was also another green sheet on top, with a hole through which the 'surgery' could be performed. On nearby shelves were a number of surgical overalls, hats, masks, gloves and overshoes. In addition, there was a set of surgical equipment.

We also had a selection of dressing-up clothes: nursing uniforms of several grades (dark blue for sister, light blue for staff nurse, green for students); a doctor's white coat, and various 'patient' outfits – pyjamas, nighties and dressing-gowns.

Procedure

The 'hospital' was set up in a spare classroom. Children were brought into the hospital in groups of three, and invited to play with the equipment for 10 minutes. Over the following month, a number of activities were organised. The children were brought back to the hospital on several occasions, by the school nurse and mother helpers. On these occasions, some of the equipment was pointed out, and ward and surgical procedures explained. Other activities included a visit to the children's ward at the local hospital, and visits to the school from an ambulance and crew, health visitor and a guide dog and owner. Each class also undertook a health-related group project.

At the second filming, children were again brought to the 'hospital' in groups of three (as before) and told that this was their last opportunity to play with the equipment before it was moved to another school. Again, their play was videotaped during the 10-minute session.

Results

Area of activity   During the first play session, most groups of children focused all their activities on the ward area, with only two groups using the surgery and one using X-ray equipment. During the second session, all groups organised their play throughout all areas of the hospital. Games were more sequenced – patients were 'admitted' to the ward, and subsequently moved to X-ray and surgery, before being discharged.

Use of equipment   Children used a range of equipment at both sessions, although at first the stethoscope, syringe, bandages and masks were used considerably more than other pieces of equipment. During the second session, there was much greater use of all the equipment, with less emphasis on the stethoscope and syringe. There were also differences in how the children used the equipment. During the first session, play was often quite rough. Children were quite aggressive in the way they gave injections, for example. On the second occasion, all children were considerably more gentle, and apparently more aware of the impact of treatment on the patient. 'Patients' were therefore likely to be warned that an injection might hurt.

'Healthcare staff' behaviour   There were substantial changes in the activities, particularly of nursing staff. During the first play session, nurses' activities involved care-taking, making beds, offering food and drink, or giving medicines. On the second, nurses spent a lot of time at the desk writing, or making phone calls. The role of the nurse seemed to have shifted from caretaker, to administrator!

Hospital atmosphere   On both occasions, children created an atmosphere of tension and emergency on the ward. Play invariably involved treating the very sick or dying, and speed and urgency characterised the interactions and conversations of staff.

Additional evaluations   All the children greatly enjoyed their time in the play hospital, and were keen to participate. Eleven children were interviewed in depth about their reactions to the project, and asked to describe what they had learned. All appeared to have benefitted substantially, both in terms of special information acquired, and in the development of non-fearful attitudes to hospital.

Does the play hospital work?

The ultimate justification for school-based preparation for hospitalisation may well be that children are less anxious and fearful about admission. There are, however, many practical difficulties involved in such an evaluation, particularly in that there may be a long interval between the intervention and admission, and that other mediating factors might then determine the child's behaviour. Such arguments have been put forward, and along with financial cuts, resulted in a reduction in these activities (Azarnoff, 1982). Certainly, the changes we identified were short-term, and we cannot speculate on the long-term value of our intervention.

Even within the short-term, however, we feel we can point to some increase in children's hospital-related knowledge. At the second session, children's play reflected greater awareness of a range of medical equipment, as well as knowledge of activities typical of admission, X-ray and surgery, and ward procedures.

There were also changes in hospital-related attitudes. The children seemed to have gained empathy with the patient's role; nurses were careful to warn patients of impending pain. In this respect, children seemed to have acquired very realistic appraisals of what happens in hospital. They were not only more aware of different equipment and techniques, but also aware of the potentially painful nature of medical treatment.

Perhaps more unfortunate was the change in children's perceptions of the nurse's role. During the first play session, 'nurses' cared for patients and tried to make them comfortable. On the second 'nurses' were preoccupied with administrative tasks, and had little, if any, time left for patient care. There also appeared to be greater awareness of a hierarchy among staff, with junior nurses being subordinate to more senior staff. To some extent, this kind of play may be closer to reality than that shown prior to the intervention, nevertheless, it seems somewhat regrettable.

Given the potential stress associated with hospitalisation (Peterson and Ridley-Johnson, 1980), it is important to develop a range of preparatory techniques for children. The school-based educational programme appears to have considerable merit, not least because it can be made available to all children before the need arises. It is not altogether clear at what level the programmes are successful; whether by increasing hospital related knowledge, reducing anxiety or helping the child develop skills to cope with hospital procedures. The success of the latter, described as 'stress-inoculation' procedures (Zastowny et al, 1986) in reducing stress in other situations (public-speaking [Cradock et al, 1978], and dental treatment [Klingman et al, 1984]), attests to the potential value of this approach in preparing children for hospitalisation.

At a practical level, the success of the play hospital is probably as dependent on the energy and enthusiasm of staff and children as on the particular contents. The overriding feeling of those who took part, however, both adults and children, was that the experience was worthwhile, and everyone learned a lot.

References

Azarnoff, P. (1982) Hospital tours for school children ended. *Pediatric Mental Health*, 1, 2.

Brett, A. (1983) Preparing children for hospitalisation – a classroom teaching approach. *Journal of School Health*, 53, 561-63.

Cradock, C., Cotler, S., Jason, L.A. (1978) Primary prevention: Immunisation of children for speech anxiety. *Cognitive Therapy and Research*, 2, 389-396.

Elkins, R. and Roberts, M. (1983) Psychological preparation for pediatric hospitalisation. *Clinical Psychology Review*, 3, 275-295.

Elkins, P. and Roberts, M. (1984) A preliminary evaluation of hospital preparation for nonpatient children: Primary prevention in a 'Let's pretend hospital'. *Children's Health Care*, 13, 31-36.

Klingman, A., Melamed, B.G., Cuthbert, M.I., Hermecz, D.A. (1984) Effects of participant modelling on information acquisition and skill utilisation. *Journal of Consulting and Clinical Psychology*, 52, 414-422.

McGarvey, M.E. (1983) Preschool hospital tours. *Children's Health Care*, 11, 122-124.

Peterson, L. and Ridley-Johnson, R. (1980) Pediatric hospital response to survey a prehospital preparation for children. *Journal of Pediatric Psychology*, 5, 1-7.

Peterson, L. and Ridley-Johnson, R. (1983) Prevention of disorders in children. In Walker, C.E. and Roberts, M.C. (Eds.) Handbook of Clinical Child Psychology. Wiley-Interscience, New York.

Roberts, M.C., Wurtele, S.K., Boone, R.R., Ginther, L.J. Elkins, P.D. (1981). Reduction of medical fears by use of modelling: A preventive application in a general population of children. *Journal of Pediatric Psychology*, 6, 293-300.

Zastowny, T.R., Kirschenbaum, D.S., Meng. A.L. (1986) Coping skills training for children: Effects on distress before, during and after hospitalisation for surgery. *Health Psychology*, 5, 231-247.

Acknowledgements

This work was funded by the Nuffield Foundation. We would like to thank Miss Joan Cudmore and the staff and children of Cowleymoor First School, Devon and Philip Gurr for technical assistance. James Lang assisted with some of the children's interviews.

7

Effective use of health education skills

Jill Macleod-Clark, PhD, BSc, SRN
Senior Lecturer in Nursing Studies, King's College, University of London

Sally Kendall, BSc, RGN, HV
Lecturer in Nursing Studies, Bucks College of Higher Education

Sheila Haverty, BA, RGN
Research Officer, Department of Nursing Studies, King's College, University of London

The importance of developing the nurse health education role is now well recognised. The need for a shift in emphasis has been accepted by the profession (UKCC,1983). Project 2000 proposals, for restructuring nurse education reflect this acceptance by recommending that health concepts and issues underpin the first eighteen months of nurse education programmes (UKCC, 1986). Similar recommendations have also been made in the Judge Report (1985) and the Cumberlege Report (1986).

There is thus a growing awareness in nursing of the need to move away from the medical model and ensure that the focus of care directed towards enhancing health. This conflict of philosophies often makes it difficult for nurses to be health educators – they are trained to care for the sick and dying by following doctors' orders not to take on a more autonomous role based on promoting or maximising health.

Previous work has shown that nurses need to develop both their knowledge and their interpersonal skills in order to become effective health educators (Faulkner and Ward, 1983; Macleod-Clark et al, 1985). It is also important that nurses have the ability to recognise opportunities for health education. Kendall has examined the opportunities nurses have in relation to smoking education (Kendall, 1986).

Smoking continues to be the largest cause of preventable disease in the UK. One in 4 of all smokers will die from a smoking related disease such as lung cancer, heart disease or chronic destructive lung disease (Doll and Peto 1981). Smoking therefore provides and excellent example of an area where nurses can develop and use their skills effectively in health education. Hopefully, it can be seen that the approach suggested is equally applicable to many other areas of health education such as nutrition and exercise.

Framework for health education

Recent research by the authors (in press) has demonstrated that health education by nurses can be effective if it is structured and skillful. The suggested framework is based on the nursing process approach since health education should be individualised like all aspects of nursing care. The long-term aim in this case is that the client stops smoking.

Assessment This involves assessing the smoker in terms of:
- Motivation to give up;
- Health beliefs and worries about smoking;
- Level of knowledge about smoking and health;
- Factors influencing smoking behaviour, eg family circumstances;
- Factual information, eg number smoked per day.

Using interpersonal skills effectively in the assessment stage is more likely to lead to an eventual successful outcome. The skills necessary for effective assessment will be discussed and illustrated with extracts from real conversations between nurses and their clients which have been recorded by the authors in the course of their research.

Questioning skills Any kind of nursing assessment requires questioning in order to gather information and to build up a complete picture of the client in terms of health and social needs. There are many ways of questioning people but two which can be most usefully employed in assessment are *open* questions and *closed* questions. Open questions usually commence with how, what, where, when, who or why. They allow the respondent to answer in their own words without limitations.

> **Example 1**
> N: How keen are you to give up?
> C: Well, I know I should give up and I know I would like to. Its just — I think it would be difficult.

Open question

In Example 1 the nurse has asked an open question in order to establish the client's level of motivation. It is important to do this in the early stages as an unmotivated client is unlikely to respond positively to any health education intervention. If the client is not motivated then the intervention should focus more on increasing motivation than changing behaviour.

Open questions are also used to find out about the client's belief system. Efforts at health education will be unsuccessful if the nurse and the client have different beliefs and values about health. If the nurse can establish what the client's beliefs are she can work within that client's frame of reference. It cannot be assumed, for example, that everybody is worried about getting lung cancer — many are not.

In Example 2 the nurse is now aware that the client is worried about breathlessness and heart disease. She could now expand on these areas

Example 2
N: What worries you about continuing
     to smoke?
C: Only that, you know, you can't
     breathe properly.
N: Mmm
C: . . . and some people get, you know,
     something wrong with their heart.

but keep the focus of her intervention on what is relevant to the client. It is equally important to establish the worries people may have about giving up smoking.

Example 3
N: What concerns you about giving up
     smoking?
C: I would really worry about putting on
     weight, there's no way I would want
     to do that.
N: Yes, a lot of women are very worried
     about that.

By asking an open question the nurse has established the client's fear of weight gain (Example 3). Obviously, this kind of information about the client is essential before any sort of plan can be formulated. This client will not feel committed to giving up smoking if she is not also given some guidance and support regarding diet and weight maintenance.

Open questions can also be used to gather factual information which will be central to the planning stage, eg "How long have you been smoking?", "How many do you smoke a day?".

Closed questions

Closed questions limit the type of response that can be given — usually to "yes" or "no". In a nursing assessment they are most useful for gathering facts quickly but should not be used to the exclusion of open questions since they do not provide the depth of information required to make a satisfactory assessment.

Example 4
N: Have you ever tried to stop smoking
     before?
C: No.

In Example 4 a simple fact has been established which may have some influence on the outcome of the intervention. For example, it is known that ex-smokers have often made several attempts to stop before they are finally successful so it would be reasonable not to expect that this client will be successful first time.

Listening and encouraging skills   Some of the most powerful skills apparently require very little effort from the nurse. However, it is more difficult than at first appears to both develop these skills and recognise their potential in assessment. Listening means more than just hearing, it means being able to interpret and make use of what is being said. In every day conversation we tend to interupt and talk over each other instead of listening. Traditionally in nursing the nurse has been very much in control of the patient which usually means she has done most of the talking. When helping people to make decisions about their lifestyle and health they should be encouraged to do the majority of the talking so that the assessment made is accurate and client-centered. Encouraging people to talk more usually only requires the nurse to give her full attention and to say things like ''uh-uh'' or ''go on''.

Example 5

N: What sort of ways have you thought about giving up smoking?

C: I've tried several times, um, and I've always stopped for about a week.

N: Mmm

C: But I get this really empty feeling inside my stomach.

N: Mmm

C: I get really moody.

N: Uh-uh

C: And I've been thinking recently, that instead of just thinking about it, I thought I'm going to set a date.

N: Mmm

C: Its best not to think about it.

As in Example 5, open questioning and encouragement often go together. By listening to this client the nurse can focus her intervention on the information she has learned.

Responding to cues Cues are hints that the client may give as to real worries not openly expressed. A skillful listener will pick up these cues and encourage the client to talk more about them. Frequently, they may be areas of concern which the client wished to discuss but was unable to — perhaps through fear, anxiety or embarrassment.

In Example 6, the nurse picks up on the client's nervousness by echoing back what the client is telling her. This technique also encourages the

Example 6

C: Um, I've been trying to cut down since I was pregnant.

N: Mmm

C: But I haven't thought about stopping altogether because it calms my nerves.

N: Mmm

C: I've been very nervous during this pregnancy.

N: You're nervous?

client to say more about the underlying cause of the nervousness so that the nurse can focus her smoking education around this, ie explore other ways of coping with anxiety.

Cues will frequently be non-verbal and it is just as important to observe and interpret these signs of anxiety and restlessness such as clock-watching or tearing up a paper handkerchief. An inattentive or worried client will not be able to respond fully to the intervention.

Giving information   During the assessment it may become apparent that there are some areas in which the client needs or requests information. Information given appropriately can enhance the client's understanding of the problem. Information given will refer back to the clients beliefs and worries and should be contained within the client's frame of reference.

Example 7
C: I think with lung cancer, I mean if your lungs pack up you have more or less had it haven't you?
N: Mmm. Yes.
C: I think that's the one that really worries me.
N: Mmm. Women are increasingly getting lung cancer because more women are smoking now. At one time, women used to think it didn't affect them and that more men die. In fact, the statistics are going up for women so it is a definite health risk.

The information given in Example 7 is appropriate because it responds to the client's worry and is given at the client's own level, avoiding jargon. Compare this with the following extract:

N: I'll just explain to you that when you smoke, carbon monoxide attaches itself to the red corpuscles that are in the blood. Blood goes to every tissue in the body so carbon monoxide, which is poison, is being sent everywhere. So what it tends to do to your hands and feet is make them tingle. Do you ever feel tingling?

C: No.

N: You don't?

C: No, never.

N: Well, this is one of the sort of circulatory problems which taken to its end is gangrene, fingers falling off and things like that.

The nurse has saturated this client with unsolicited and inappropriate information. She has used technical terms which may mean nothing to the client and has resorted to terror tactics to gain her client's attention. It is not necessary to tell every client everything you know about smoking.

Where information is given it is often useful to back it up with written material so that the client has a chance to absorb the information quietly

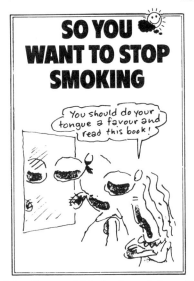

It is often useful to back up information with written material such as this HEA leaflet.

later on. There are many leaflets and booklets freely available on smoking and other subjects from health education units.

In summary, the initial assessment involves the skills of questioning, listening, encouraging, responding to cues and giving appropriate information. The aim of the assessment is to build up a picture of the client, enabling the nurse to focus her intervention within the client's frame of reference.

Planning

When formulating a plan the overall aim should be kept in sight, ie cessation of smoking. However, before a total behaviour change is achieved there may be other short term goals to be met. Such short term goals should be realistic and mutually agreed between the client and the nurse. Frequently, the client may be pleased to accept the nurse's guidance as she will have practical suggestions and access to methods of cessation (see Kendall, 1986) previously unavailable or unknown to the client. However, a plan conceived and imposed by the nurse alone is unlikely to be successful. Some short term goals which may be useful to consider are:

- Create no-smoking areas in the home/car;
- Keep a smoking diary for one week, ie write down how many cigarettes are smoked, when and why;
- Reduce smoking by half within one week;
- Find out where the nearest smokers clinic is.

The overall plan and the short term goals should be based on the needs and beliefs established during the assessment. For example, if a client smokes as a way of relieving stress then the plan should be based on alternative methods of coping with stress. Asking questions such as "How do you think you could go about giving up?" may be useful in giving some initial direction to the plan and in helping the client to feel that she is participating in the lifestyle changes she is making.

Clients often feel that a behaviour such as smoking is outside their control and that the risks of smoking are on a par with the risks of nuclear war for example. Clients should be helped to see that they can control their own behaviour and setting realistic goals often helps to put the behaviour into perspective.

Implementation

Once the client and the nurse have established the "giving up" plan in which there are agreed goals and objectives it is up to the client to implement it. Many smokers will say "It is only me that can do it". This is true, but the client can be helped by offering support. This could be done in the form of leaving a telephone number on which the nurse could be contacted (eg on the ward or health centre) or could be more formalised with future meetings being planned. If it is inappropriate for the nurse herself to offer support (ward-based nurses may find this difficult) then support could be sought from within the family or friendship network. For example, partners may find it helpful to give up together. Some clients might be attracted to group support and in this case a stop smoking group may be appropriate. Whatever form the support takes it must suit both the client and the nurse.

Evaluation

Whenever possible, following an intervention the nurse should arrange to see the client again at least once. This could take place in the home, in the antenatal clinic, outpatients clinic or wherever is most appropriate to the nurse's field of work. This follow-up has a dual purpose. It gives the client something to work towards and allows priorities to be reorganised and goals reset.

If, by the time of the agreed follow-up, there has been no demonstrable change in behaviour, the nurse should not regard her intervention as a complete failure. Many ex-smokers make several attempts before finally giving up and a change in motivation is as successful as a change in behaviour. It may be that the continued interest and support of the nurse will give the smoker the required impetus to give up eventually.

However, a reassessment of the previous intervention will give guidance for tackling problems and setting new short-term goals. If the original plan was unsuccessful it may be necessary to make adjustments or formulate a new one. If the client is successful in giving up smoking then she should be encouraged to continue and where possible continued support offered if required.

In summary, this framework requires the nurse to assess her client, make a plan of action with the client, support and encourage the client in its implementation and evaluate the intervention.

It may at first appear that the framework is complicated and time consuming. However, in their research the authors have found that with practice, it is possible to assess and plan in five to 10 minutes. The framework aims to be flexible and adaptable to various work settings. For example, if ward based nurses find the idea of giving continued support unrealistic due to high turnover of patients then they could either give the client their ward telephone number or refer her/him to one of their community colleagues. Health visitors and district nurses will have more prolonged contact with their clients and may decide to spread the assessment and planning over two visits and they will be more able to offer support over a period of time.

The framework is not rigid and if nurses of all disciplines could adapt it and use it in their every day practise there is potential for a considerable impact on attaining the WHO target of health for all by the year 2000.

References

Cumberlege, J. et al (1986) Neighbourhood nursing – a focus for care. Report of the Community Nursing Review. HMSO. London.

Doll, R. and Peto, R. (1981) The Causes of Cancer. Oxford University Press.

Faulkner, A and Ward L (1983) Nurses as health educators in relation to smoking, *Nursing Times*, Occasional Paper 8, **79**, 15, 47-48.

Kendall, S. (1986) Helping people to stop smoking. *The Professional Nurse*, **1**, 5, 120-123.

Macleod-Clark, J. Elliot, K. Haverty, S. and Kendall, S. (1985) Helping people to stop smoking – the nurse's role. Phase 1. Health Education Council, London.

Macleod-Clark, J. Haverty, S. and Kendall, S. (1987) Helping people to stop smoking – the nurse's role. Research Report No.19.

Judge, H. et al (1985) Commission on nurse education. RCN, London.

United Kingdom Central Council for Nurses, Midwives and Health Visitors. (1986) Project 2000, UKCC.

World Health Organisation (1978) Report of an international conference on primary health care Alma-Ata, USSR. WHO, Geneva.

8

Educating patients at home

Pauline Bagnall, SRN
Angela Heslop, DipN(Lond) RCNT SRN
Research Fellows, Department of Medicine, Charing Cross and Westminster Medical School, London

Teaching involves application of good communication skills, and the outcome can have dramatic and positive effects on the quality of life and wellbeing of patients, particularly those whose illness or disability is long-term. This chapter outlines a study which was undertaken to assess the value of educating patients with chronic respiratory disease about their condition.

Recommendation

Chronic respiratory disease is an important cause of disability, a fact recently recognised in a report from the Royal College of Physicians (1981). It recommended that a Respiratory Health Worker (RHW) should be appointed on a trial basis to visit and care for people suffering from chronic lung disease at home.

A controlled trial, to evaluate the effect of RHWs, was undertaken in 1984 (Cockcroft et al, 1986). Seventy-five patients were randomised to one of two groups: 42 patients to the intervention group (visited by the RHW) and 33 patients to the control group.

The aims of the study were to improve the patients' quality of life and to reduce their hospital admissions. Two nurses, (the authors) with experience of looking after people with chest disease were employed to fill the Respiratory Health Worker post. In addition one had experience of working in the community. People were visited approximately monthly, intervention being mainly preventive, supportive and educative.

Methods

The Royal College of Physicians' Report suggested that one role of the RHW might be 'promoting respiratory health education and practices' (Royal College of Physicians, 1981). In our study both the intervention and the control group completed questionnaires at the beginning and end of the study year. There were specific questions about knowledge of condition and medicines, as well as questions about smoking habits and activities of daily living. Our brief was to be educators and we knew that the patient's education was to be a measured outcome of the research.

We concentrated on the individuality of the patient, using Roper's model (Roper et al, 1983) incorporating a problem solving approach. On the first visit we assessed the patient in terms of daily living activities and knowledge of chest disease and medicines. For example, was it known what the illness was called, how it affected the patient and what the names and actions of the medicines were? From this first assessment problems would be identified and goals set. On each subsequent visit we would evaluate the patient's progress and redefine goals as appropriate.

Education programme

Most patients in the study had not been expected to learn about their disease or medicines before. Many had left school at an early age and so to learn was a new experience. They had other health problems besides chest disease such as poor eyesight, impaired hearing and other illnesses. They had also lost loved ones and a sense of worth. When deciding how to structure the teaching programme all these factors had to be taken into account.

We worked with each individual in his/her home; tailoring the teaching to his/her needs. However a basic format did emerge. From the initial assessment on the first visit areas of knowledge which were lacking would be identified. It was first established that medicines were being taken as prescribed. If this was not so it was corrected and explanations were given about the appropriate use of medicines. Another priority was to establish if the patient knew how to recognise deterioration in lung disease (usually secondary to infection) and in this event what action to take. Gradually over the course of the year each patient's knowledge of his illness and management increased as he was able to assimilate information about anatomy and physiology of the heart and lungs and names and actions of his medicines.

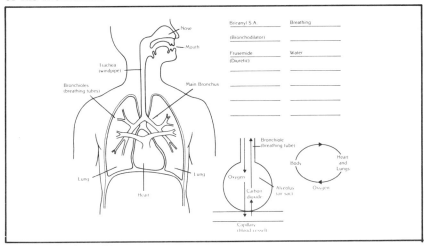

Figure 1. Teaching aid.

A teaching aid (Figure 1) was designed and given to each patient to keep. It was used to present facts visually with colours. The information was given in simple terms with both anatomical and colloquial names used. For example, the lungs were often described as being analogous to sponges with blue blood going in and red blood coming out; the bronchi were often referred to as breathing tubes. Where possible Health Education Council pamphlets about diet and smoking supplemented the teaching. The aim was to increase the patient's understanding of his disease and of how to cope with particular problems.

Date	Problem	Goal LT-long term, ST-short term.	Care Plan	Date	Evaluation
1st visit	Mr L is unable to recognise deterioration in his lung disease.	**LT** Mr L will tell me at the end of the year the significance of discoloured sputum and the action to be taken. **ST** Mr L will tell me next visit what colour sputum should be, what green/yellow sputum may indicate and what he will do if this occurs.	Explain to Mr L the importance of green/yellow sputum and that a chest infection may be present. Tell him to call his GP should this occur.	2nd visit	Mr L told me his sputum should be white and that green/yellow sputum indicates a chest infection is present when he will call his GP.
2nd visit	Mr L does not check the colour of his sputum every day.	**ST** Mr L is to tell me that antibiotics will be prescribed by the GP for a chest infection, that the full course should be taken and if he is not better he is to contact his GP again. He is to check the colour of his sputum daily.	Explain to Mr L why it is important to check his sputum every day. Explain about antibiotics.	3rd visit	Mr L told me antibiotics will be prescribed for a chest infection and it is important to finish the whole course. He also said he will contact his GP again if he is no better and that he checks his sputum daily.
3rd visit	Mr L does not have a reserve supply of antibiotics at home.	**ST** Mr L is to ask his GP for a reserve supply of antibiotics to keep at home. He is to start a course if his sputum changes colour, complete the course and contact the GP if he is no better. He is to tell me next visit how many times a day he takes the antibiotics and for how long.	Explain about the role of reserve antibiotics.	4th visit	Mr L told me he did get a reserve supply of antibiotics from his GP and had commenced a course 3 days ago because his sputum became green. He is taking 1 tablet 3 x a day for 7 days. He will get another reserve supply when this course is completed.

Table 2. Part of the education programme for Mr L.

Table 2 illustrates part of one patient's teaching programme. Mr L is a 59 year old man with chronic obstructive airways disease. On the first visit it was established that he continued to smoke, did not know how to detect deterioration in his lung disease and did not know the names or actions of his medicines. From this example it can be seen that gradually the knowledge base was built up so that Mr L became responsible for this aspect of his own health and confident in caring for himself. A similar plan was used to help him stop smoking and learn about his disease and medicines.

Education was not only confined to these areas. Some patients were overweight in which case advice about diet and the use of weight charts was given. Other patients were underweight and required some simple cooking lessons. Improving mobility was another major area of our work. Some patients enjoyed programmes to increase their activity. For example, one lady wanted to walk to the library to change her books. We started a training programme in which she started walking around her flat more often; this was gradually extended to walking outside to the rubbish shute every day and eventually she reached her stated goal which was the library. It was important to acknowledge the progress made with encouragement and congratulation.

Patients' response

Most patients wanted to learn more about their disease and medicines. We structured our work on individual patient care so that they were taught as much or as little as they wanted to know. Some found it difficult to retain information, in which case the priority was to make certain that medicines were being taken correctly and that the patient could act appropriately on signs of deterioration. Others wanted to have more detailed knowledge about how the heart and lungs interact and the way in which their medicines acted. An important point to remember was that on some visits education was not of primary importance to the person concerned. In one instance a lady's budgerigar — her 'companion' — had died the previous day. It would have been inappropriate to talk about her medicines when she wanted to talk about her grief. Some of the patients 'prepared' for our visits. One man said he always looked at his list of medicines before a visit because he knew he would be asked about them. Other patients had their medicines on the table ready. Nearly all said that they had valued the time to learn, the individual teaching they received and the opportunity to ask questions. Most importantly, they valued the knowledge which enabled them to look after themselves.

Effectiveness of the programme

The questionnaire replies about knowledge of condition and medicines were evaluated by two physicians not involved in the study. Knowledge was scored as being either poor, adequate or good and an assessment was made of whether knowledge had improved, remained the same or become worse over the course of the year. There was no significant difference between the groups in their knowledge of their condition or medicines at the beginning of the study. At the end of the study significantly more people in the RHW group than in the control group had improved their knowledge of their condition (combined X^2 5.62,

Changes during the study	RHW Group	Control Group
Physician 1		
Number with Worse	3	2
knowledge: The same	15	15
Better	14	6
Physician 2		
Number with Worse	3	0
knowledge: The same	15	19
Better	14	4

Table 3: Knowledge of condition as assessed by two independent physicians, based on questionnaire answers.

p<0.05)(Table 3) and a similar trend was seen for knowledge of medicines.

The teaching programme was goal directed. Of the education goals set, more than 75 per cent were considered by the RHWs to have been achieved by the patients concerned.

Personal experience of the project

Before I (Pauline Bagnall) joined the research project my teaching experience was limited to a teaching exercise I did during the Cardiothoracic Nursing Course ENB 249 and a few short sessions I gave to nurses on the ward. I had not been involved with teaching patients. I spent much time discussing with my colleague how we would approach the teaching aspect of our new role. We were aware that our patients would be elderly and that education might be a new experience for them. I was also aware that this was 'research' and that my work was being monitored and measured. I therefore wanted my patients to learn.

Initially I was shocked at how little knowledge these people had and therefore tried to give them too much information all at once. Gradually I learned to give only as much information as the patient wanted or needed. I also learned to give the information in order of priority — making sure the patient was safe.

Several insights came to me as a result of my participation in this work. I realised that all my patients were chronically ill at home and they had all learned to cope and adapt to their problems in a variety of ways. I had previously only nursed people in hospital where it is difficult to visualise how someone manages at home in a tiny house rather than in a big new hospital. Another insight arose because I was visiting patients in their homes where they not I were in control. I also had no hospital routine or uniform to support me. I had only my personality and expertise to offer. For the first time I felt truly accountable for what I was doing. I was visiting a patient in his home independently and over the course of a year I had a responsibility to help him to cope with his disability. I learned to value my role as a nurse and at the same time to respect each patient as an individual person.

Education needs

It has been recognised that patients need to have information, and guidance to understand this information in order to care for themselves (Redman, 1981). It is also known that understanding their disease and medicines improves patient compliance (Weibert and Dee, 1980). There has been an increasing interest in patient education since the early 1970s and most writers support the idea that nurses should teach patients (Cohen, 1981). Yet, in 1985 Wilson-Barnett published a paper saying that despite all the evidence "when nurses are questioned they accept that patients' information needs are not met" (Wilson-Barnett, 1985).

There seem to be many reasons for this lack of teaching. Wilson-Barnett goes on to say that "teaching does not occur because nurses are inadequately qualified'' (Wilson-Barnett, 1985). Learning to teach is not a defined subject in the curriculum for nurse registration. Nurses on average spend only 10 per cent of their time communicating with patients (Macleod Clark, 1983) yet the few studies that have addressed the function of nurses as health educators have all concluded that such patient/client teaching as is done, is done by nurses (Gleit and Graham, 1984).

An important aspect of the research was our role as educators. The results confirm that our patients did learn more about their disease and medicines and how to cope with their disability. The reasons for this success are many. The teaching programme took place in the patient's home which seemed to produce a more conducive atmosphere both for teaching and learning than the busy, noisy hospital. Whenever possible the family also learned and therefore supported the patient. The information was given in small measures and repeated if necessary. This opportunity for repetition and recall helped the patient to fully understand before moving on. Continuity of the visits and the development of a relationship sustained for six-to-nine months was important in the learning process. The patient learned to trust us and felt able to talk about problems he may not have mentioned before.

All the patients were attending the Department of Medicine of a large teaching hospital and had suffered from chronic lung disease for many years. They had all been in hospital several times, yet their knowledge at the beginning of the study was very poor. There is clearly a need to introduce teaching programmes in hospital before discharge, to be continued by community nurses at home. It is the experience of other authors (Wilson-Barnett, 1983; Nuffield Working Party, 1980) and our own experience in this study that patients do want to know more and nurses may be the appropriate people to teach them. We believe it will be beneficial for nurses to know that their work has enabled patients to become more confident and able to take care of themselves.

Acknowledgements
We are grateful to Dr A. Cockcroft and Professor A. Guz, Department of Medicine, Charing Cross and Westminster Medical School, for their advice and support.

References
Cockcroft, A., Bagnall, P., Heslop, A. et al (1986) Controlled trial of a respiratory health worker visiting patients with chronic respiratory disability. Submitted to the *British Medical Journal*. **294**, 225-7.
Cohen, S.A. (1981) Patient Education: a review of the literature. *Journal of Advanced Nursing*, **6**, 1, 11-18.
Gleit, C.J., Graham, B.A. (1984) Reading materials used in the preparation of nurses for the teaching role. *Patient Education and Counselling*, **6**, 1, 25-28.
Macleod-Clark J. (1983) Nurse patient communication – an analysis of conversations from surgical wards. In: Wilson-Barnett, J., (Ed), Nursing Research: Ten studies in Patient Care, Wiley, Chichester.
Nuffield Working Party (1980) Talking with Patients: A Teaching Approach, Nuffield, Provincial Hospitals Trust.
Redman, B.K. (1981) Issues and Concepts in Patient Education, Appleton-Century-Crofts, New York.

Roper, N., Logan, W., Tierney, A.J. (1983). Using a model for nursing, Churchill-Livingstone, Edinburgh.

Royal College of Physicians (1981) Disabling Chest Disease: Prevention and care. *Journal of the Royal College of Physicians of London*, **15**, 2, 69-87.

Weibert, R.T., Dee, D.A. (1980) Improving Patient Medication Compliance 1, Medical Economics Company, New Jersey.

Wilson-Barnett, J., Osborne, J. (1983) Studies evaluating patient teaching: implications for practice. *International Journal of Nursing Studies*, **20**, 1, 33-44.

Wilson-Barnett, J. (1985) Principles of patient teaching. *Nursing Times*, **81**, 8, 28-29.

9

Communication can help ostomists accept their stoma

Ian Donaldson, RGN DIPN
Currently studying for a BEd (Nursing) at the Polytechnic of the South Bank, London.

Throughout this chapter, for reasons of conciseness, the female gender has been used to describe nurses of either gender and the male to describe patients of either gender.

Ward based nurses can play an important part in helping ostomists to adapt to their new situation, enabling them to reintegrate into society. Many wards do not have access to the services of a full time stoma therapist, and so general nurses need to be able to care for and assist ostomists. A recent study showed that many nurses feel unprepared for the complexities of stoma care (Monnington, 1987), so ostomists on their wards are likely to have little preparation for their future life.

In most cases, the formation of a stoma is life improving (eg, ulcerative colitis) or life saving (eg, perforated diverticulum). Some surgeons regard stoma formation for cancer as life saving, but this disregards the patient's expectation of the diagnosis of cancer, which to most people means unpleasant death (Broardwell and Jackson, 1982).

Devlin (1985) refers to ostomists as "people who have traded death for disablement", and this hints at the profound effect this type of surgery has on the individual. Society values health as desirable but its picture of health is of someone who has total control over bodily functions and is odour free. The formation of a stoma removes the patient's ability to control elimination and presents the possibility of leakage or release of flatus in any situation, a similar picture to an incontinent person. Fear of rejection by family and friends due to stigma is particularly acute, so new ostomists have to face many problems and anxieties before they feel able to return to their previous social situation (Kelly, 1985).

Preoperative care

It is useful to consider preoperative care under the two broad headings of physical and psychological. As with general surgery, physical preparation is usually carried out effectively, but it is important that issues such as siting the stoma are dealt with. An incorrectly sited stoma can cause much distress and may reduce the ostomist's ability to cope with the stoma in the future. The type of clothing the patient wears, skin creases and his ability to reach and see the site must be considered. Some ethnic groups have been reported to accept their stoma better if it is sited above the umbilicus, as the discharge is then associated with clean food contained in the stomach rather than bowel contents (Whitethread, 1981). It is also important to take into consideration the ostomist's cultural/ spiritual background for other reasons. For example, the concept of cleanliness is very important to Muslims; faeces are considered unclean and so a stoma will present a Muslim with difficult problems. The requirement that he is 'clean' before prayer will mean frequent appliance changes, similarly his right hand should be kept clean and should not handle faeces. This obviously will present great difficulties to any Muslim trying to change his appliance one handed. Difficulties like this can greatly inhibit acceptance of a stoma, and it is important that the nurse is aware of these as potential problems and is prepared to support the patient.

Many studies have indicated that preoperative information giving and visits reduce anxiety, which is not only beneficial for the patient, but also for the nurse. Anxiety has been recognised as a barrier to learning, so it is of great advantage to have a less anxious patient postoperatively. Sadly, this area of patient care is all too often neglected. It is important for the nurse to assess what the patient is aware of and be prepared to put right any misconceptions he may have. Both nurses and doctors are much to blame for giving inadequate information. How often have we heard or used the phrase "don't worry its only a little bag on your tummy". Are these the reassuring words we should be using? Ridgeway and Matthews (1983) describe a method called cognitive coping, in which the patient is encouraged to identify fears and anxieties about the operation and its after effects to the nurse and to highlight the areas in which he is most concerned. The nurse and the patient then deal with these fears, either by presenting them in a positive light or dealing with any misconceptions. This positive reappraisal involves an altered perception of the threatening situation; the nurse provides the patient with accurate information that he can understand, and which he can use to cope with the impending situation. For example, a patient with colitis who is about to have a permament ileostomy may be helped to reflect on the fact that afterwards he will not have to repeatedly come back to hospital due to remissions, and his health will improve. A patient who has just been told he needs a colostomy due to a perforated diverticulum will be greatly relieved to hear this type of surgery is life saving and the stoma is usually only temporary. It has to be accepted however that patients are often sceptical of information and need to see the evidence. Associations such as the Ileostomy Association can provide visitors, who are ostomists themselves, and can show the patient that normal life after- wards is possible. Care must be taken, however, to ensure the 'visitor' is experienced and a suitable role model. Most ostomists' postoperative problems can be placed in two groups; physical and psychosocial, and both are of importance when planning appropriate care.

Physical care

It is useful to note that the patient's ability to change his appliance is usually, (though not always) the criteria used for discharge, so it is an important nursing aim to assist the patient to be responsible for his own self-care actions (Orem, 1985). Inherent in this statement is that the nurse is an educator. Orem breaks down self-care deficits (inability to care for oneself) into three areas: knowledge, skill, and motivation. It is useful for the nurse to consider these areas when planning care. To give self-care, the ostomist needs the necessary knowledge and skills to care for the stoma on a daily basis, and will need to develop skills related to changing his appliance (when and how to change), and knowledge as to how to obtain, store and dispose of the appliances. He will also need to learn about diet, skin care, how to deal with problems such as leaks, skin excoriation, odour and flatus and when to seek medical advice.

The nurse should be constantly aware that she is teaching the patient, so he can return to his home and normal activities. Many patients will return to houses without inside toilets; similarly, one who wishes to return to work as a travelling salesman will need to be able to deal with his stoma in a variety of settings. Awareness of what the patient is intending to return to is obviously important.

When planning the patient's care with him, it is important that realistic goals are negotiated and set. The patient is likely to become despondent if he is told "don't worry we'll have you managing this next week" and next week arrives and he has not been able yet to master emptying his appliance. However, if realistic short term goals are set (eg, will be able to apply clip to drainable appliance), when they are met the patient will feel a sense of achievement. Using short term goals as building blocks allows the patient to progress at his speed and can also be used to show him that he *is* making progress.

The right environment

When teaching the patient the nurse must ensure that the right learning environment is created. It is absolutely no use to try and teach someone who is in pain or tired. Showing the patient equipment and using diagrams can be useful, and it is vital that the nurse avoids using jargon. If the patient does not understand he may not ask and so will not learn. An important aspect of teaching is to assess what the patient has actually learnt. All too often it seems nurses believe that if they have told the patient what to do then he will do it. The patient's level of comprehension must be assessed – it is not enough just to give information and expect the patient to act on it, and recall of information does not necessarily mean that the patient comprehends it. Comprehension is vital if the patient is to apply this knowledge to solving new problems he may encounter.

Psychosocial care

As already mentioned, stoma formation has an immense impact on the

patient's psychological and sociological wellbeing. Most patients suffer from low self-esteem postoperatively, usually due to altered body image. The patient's level of self-esteem is a result of evaluation of his self concept, of which his body image is a part. Body image is 'how we see ourselves', and includes not only our physical appearance but also our beliefs, goals and other people's opinions of us. According to Meisenhelder (1985) the perceived respect, love and approval of people close to us (significant others) have a considerable effect on our self-esteem. She suggests three groups of people who can raise the patient's self-esteem:
• other patients in a similar situation;
• family and friends (significant others);
• nursing and other medical staff.

As patients do not stay in hospital for any great length of time, they don't often get the opportunity to meet others in a similar situation. However, self help groups can be beneficial to the patient as they allow him to meet others in a similar situation to him with whom he can talk and discuss problems. A fellow ostomist is unlikely to give him a negative appraisal or avoid him, and this will therefore create an atmosphere conducive to raising his self-esteem. He may also be able to obtain practical advice that will be useful in future.

In the postoperative period the patient will be testing his family and friends to find their response to his stoma. Their acceptance of the stoma is a major help towards the patient's sucessful adaption to the stoma (Broardwell and Jackson, 1982). He will use their responses as predictors of future interactions with other people, so a negative appraisal (actual or perceived) from the patient's significant others will only confirm his fears that he has become a social outcast. The nurse can help by preparing and supporting family and friends so they can help raise the patient's self-esteem and increase the likelihood of his acceptance of the stoma.

According to Porrit (1984) the nurse can raise the patient's self-esteem by effectively communicating a sense of worth and value for the patient, showing that he is truly valued as a human being. This can be achieved through touch and reflective listening, an approach she calls 'unconditional positive regard' through which the nurse can help the patient explore his feelings and fears without judgement.

Ostomists fear rejection by others and worry about how they will relate to them. If this fear becomes all consuming, the ostomist may retreat from social contact. Studies have shown (Devlin, 1971; MacDonald and Anderson, 1984) that many ostomists retreat from social life. Nurses can help them cope with any insecurities they may face due to their attempt to reintegrate back into society. Price (1986) suggests a framework for this (Table 1) which gives patients three possible approaches to use. Preparation of these responses can give them confidence when meeting people who know they have been in hospital. By using simple interventions like those discussed in this chapter, nurses can assist ostomists greatly in accepting their stomas.

POSSIBLE APPROACH USED			
Relevant person.	OPEN FRANK.	MODIFIED FRANK.	RESTRICTED.
Spouse.	✓		
Children.		✓	
Close colleagues	✓		
Other colleagues.			✓
Close relative.		✓	
Distant relatives.			✓

Table 1. A framework for reintegration. **Open frank:** *explanation showing of new image, equipment and aids. Recognition and comment made upon aetiology and prognosis as understood. Frank expression of how new image makes you feel.* **Modified frank:** *Explanation of current physical shape/image but not showing actual part of body that is changed. Indicate how you feel in general terms. No comment on aetiology or implications for the future.* **Restricted:** *Indication that operation has taken place but no direct reference to new image.*

References

Broardwell, D. and Jackson, B. (1982) Principles of Ostomy Care. C.V. Mosby, London.

Devlin, B. (1985) Second opinion. *Health and Social Services Journal*, **95**, 4931, 82.

Devlin, B. et al (1971) Aftermath of surgery for anorectal cancer. *British Medical Journal*, **3**, 413-418.

Kelly, M. (1985) Loss and grief reactions as a response to surgery. *Journal of Advanced Nursing*, **10**, 517-525.

Meisenhelder, J. (1985) Self-Esteem: A closer look at clinical interventions. *International Journal of Nursing Studies*. **22**, 2, 127-135.

Monnington, M. (1987) Teaching and counselling support for new stoma patients – a survey of the views of patients and trained nurses. Unpublished MSc thesis. Kings College, London.

Macdonald, L. and Anderson, H. (1984) Stigma in patients with rectal cancer: A community study. *Journal of Epidemology and Community Health*, **38**, 284-290.

Orem, D. (1985) Nursing: Concepts of Practice. Mcgraw Hill, New York.

Porrit, L. (1984) Communication: Choices for Nurses. Churchill Livingstone, London.

Price, B. (1986) Keeping up appearances. *Nursing Times*, **82**, 40, 58-61.

Ridgeway, V. and Matthews, A. (1982) Psychological preparation for surgery: A comparison of methods. *British Journal of Psychology*, **21**, 271-280.

Whitethread, M. (1981) Ostomists; A world of difference. *Journal of Community Nursing*, **5**, 2, 4-10.

Counselling

10

Introducing nurses to the counselling process

Patrick McEvoy, RMN, SRN, DipN, RCNT, RNT

Senior Tutor, Department of Postbasic Education, College of Mental Health Nursing, Belfast

"Counselling is a personal relationship in which the counsellor uses his own experiences of himself to help his client to enlarge his self-understanding and so make better decisions" (Sutherland, 1973).

"Counselling is a relationship in which one person endeavours to help another to understand and solve the difficulties of adjustment to society" (Heasman, 1969).

"Counselling gives a person the opportunity to discover, explore and clarify ways of living more resourcefully and towards greater well-being" (British Association of Counselling, 1979).

Counselling is a complex process which is difficult to define, never mind teach, as the definitions above indicate. For this reason some people will say such teaching should be left to the professional counsellor, as student nurses may become confused with a concept which is open to so many interpretations.

In the context of nursing, however, I would suggest a simple definition of the concept: "Counselling is an enabling interaction between two people which seeks to support the weaker person as a responsible human being". Within this definition it is difficult to visualise a situation whereby a nurse would care for patients' daily needs and yet avoid involvement in counselling – a nurse cannot provide care without counselling. She does not really have a choice. Patients will inevitably bring their problems to her and she will be expected to counsel as part of her role. In this respect she must frequently respond to the unexpected, whereas full time counsellors work in much more structured situations. The nurse's choice, then, is between counselling in a competent and informed manner or in a haphazard thoughtless fashion. All nurses should therefore be properly introduced to the counselling process at an early stage in their training. Counselling competence, however, cannot be achieved through a one-off experience at the beginning of a nurse's education. Rather, it must weave into her professional fabric throughout her professional life supported by a sound programme of continuing education.

Presenting the skills

Counselling skills need to be presented in such a way that nurses will immediately grasp their relevance to nursing. Initially their interest must be aroused by drawing attention to the problems they will be confronted with in the clinical setting and offering to help find some of the answers. It is useful to give them first hand accounts of counselling situations which develop in the hospital wards. The following points can be emphasised:

- Nurses spend more time with patients than any other health professionals.
- The social distance is least between the patient and the nurse. Therefore it is likely that the patient will feel that he can confide in the nurse more than in anyone else.
- Virtually all ill people have problems which may be amenable to counselling.
- All nurses counsel patients. In many instances counselling is integral to the provision of care; for example, even helping a patient to feel at home in hospital may involve counselling.

Having established that counselling is intrinsically linked with the provision of care, nurses should be placed in small groups and encouraged to discuss their own ideas of counselling. To correct misconceptions, the facilitator must circulate from group to group and make certain all individuals are aware of a simple definition like the one previously mentioned: "Counselling is an enabling interaction between two people which seeks to support the weaker person as a responsible human being". Counselling must never be confused with simply giving advice.

Offering help

Counselling involves one person offering to help another. No-one can help another without at least having begun to understand that person, and one cannot begin to understand others until one understands oneself, so nurses must be aware that effective counselling is unlikely to occur without self-knowledge. It is most unwise for anyone involved in counselling to ignore her own feelings, needs and problems.

The process of self-disclosure can be stimulated by asking each nurse to pair off with someone she does not know intimately and engage in a mutual exchange of personal information. When the pairs have been together for about 10 minutes the tutor should ask couples to become foursomes and repeat the exercise. At this stage the tutor might present each group with some light and amusing topic to discuss such as 'what would you do if a kissogram girl/boy called for you?' Such topics reduce self-consciousness and encourage spontaneity; and it is remarkable how they frequently develop into serious discussion around ethical matters like sexism and sexual behaviour in general. Having broken the ice during these preliminary exercises, nurses can move more confidently into discussion of their own self-awareness in relation to counselling.

Self-awareness includes self-image – how you see yourself; and self-esteem – how you think others see you. Some young people come into nursing with poor self-esteem, and it is essential that this is detected before they move into situations where they will attempt to counsel others. They must be encouraged to be more self-revealing than self-concealing. The facilitator must always be available to listen to nurses talking about their problems, and be willing to help them develop on their own terms. A nurse lacking in self-esteem will very soon get out of her depth in the mental health field. Not all patients will be honest and cooperative. Some will exhibit conscious or unconscious desires to manipulate and frustrate those who offer to help them. Such patients can be adept at getting their own way through covert manipulation. Student nurses are particularly vulnerable. Not wishing to be labelled like "that other insensitive nurse who didn't understand", the inexperienced nurse may be too eager to be helpful. She must know there will always be someone to whom she can turn for support; someone who will enable her to ask herself questions like, "Am I being taken beyond my responsibilities as a nurse?", and "What does this patient really want?"

Attitude of the counsellor

Unhealthy attitudes on the part of nurses can also inhibit counselling. Research has clearly indicated that counselling is only successful when the counsellor displays warmth, sensitivity and understanding, and is willing to meet patients with an open attitude. Relationship is infinitely more important than technique. Successful counsellors radiate sincerity and are able to confront in a constructive manner. Of course, not all nurses will possess these qualities, but they must be made aware of the desirability of developing their personalities along these lines if they are to help patients cope with their problems.

As the facilitator discusses these matters with nurses, she should pay particularly attention to individuals who express reservations about these ideas, for their defence mechanisms may be rejecting some aspects of counselling, for example self-disclosure, on emotional grounds. On the other hand, it may be that the concepts have not been sufficiently explained. Since counselling is based on ideas borrowed from other disciplines such as philosophy, psychiatry and theology, different meanings may become attached to words, with consequent confusion.

Counselling concepts are difficult to comprehend in the abstract and for ethical reasons cannot be freely tested with patients, so nurses must be placed in simulated situations which will enable them to get the feel of the skills involved. Three or four of the basic components of counselling should be isolated, and structured opportunities created for the students to practise them. This is usually the prerogative of the facilitator. I would propose the following skills to begin with; attending, listening, leading and demonstrating empathy. More difficult skills such as summarising, reflecting and confronting may be introduced as the nurse gains experience.

Attending   This is the giving of undivided attention to the patient who seeks help through:
- eye contact – looking (without staring) in such a way as to communicate concern and understanding;
- a posture which is relaxed and focused towards the patient;
- gestures and facial expressions which are natural, but not excessive or distracting.

Listening   "If one gives answer before he hears, it is his folly and shame", (Proverbs 18:13). My favourite definition of listening is "not thinking about what you are going to say until the other person has stopped talking". Many people fail to listen because they are already concentrating on what they wish to say in response. Waiting through periods of silence as the patient summons up courage to delve into painful memories, or pauses to collect his thoughts can be tedious and tiresome, yet nothing destroys counselling as much as excessive talking by the counsellor. A nurse who talks a lot to patients may give good advice, but this is seldom heard and even less likely to be acted on. Listening is one of the most effective ways of caring.

Nurses must be made aware that if they find themselves talking a lot to patients, this may be an expression of their own insecurities. They may feel unable to handle situations which they don't fully understand or find too emotional or threatening. If so, they should be advised to withdraw and seek help from more experienced people. Listening is essentially a sensitive monitoring of the other person's words to try to understand his perceived problems and underlying emotions.

Leading   Despite the emphasis on listening as the core of counselling, the patient must obviously be asked some questions, but how? Questions should be simply phrased and asked one at a time, avoiding those which can be answered by a simple yes or no. Questions involving the use of the word 'why' are also undesirable since they may appear too judgmental. Open-ended questions such as; "You said a few minutes ago that you have been having difficulties at work. Tell me a bit more about this?" are far preferable. The judicious use of questions can gently lead the patient into productive channels of exploration. The competent counsellor will ask the patient those questions which he should be asking of himself. Subtle questioning can also help the patient inject a sense of order and perspective into his life situation.

Demonstrating empathy   This is the ability to demonstrate to a person that you can view the situation from his point of view. It is vital that nurses can clearly distinguish between empathy and sympathy. Empathy is to understand the feelings of another person; sympathy is being affected yourself by the same feelings experienced by the other person, and is a hidden danger for the inexperienced nurse. Empathy embraces the ability of the counsellor to remain impartial and not allow her own feelings to intrude into the counselling situation. It is an elusive quality which cannot always be conjured up because it seems the right way to feel. It is related to experience. The closer the nurse's own life experience to that of the patient the more likely she is to understand how the patient feels. On the other hand, sympathy can easily replace empathy if the nurse becomes over-involved with an individual's problems.

The success of any attempt to teach counselling is closely related to the graded presentation of the relevant skills together with a plan to teach them in an interesting and purposeful manner. I have always found simple, direct person-to-person methods most effective. Using a battery of media, including closed circuit TV, tapes and films can be distracting and confusing for students and facilitator alike. Role play supported by group discussion is obviously the medium of choice.

To facilitate this approach, an easy relationship between facilitator and nurse is essential. There must be a considerable degree of mutual trust and acceptance. Initially the role model must be willing to demonstrate the skills herself. Lack of finesse need not be a drawback. A highly skilled model may actually increase performance anxiety in nurses, whereas a model who copes in spite of shortcomings will encourage nurses to launch out themselves.

Having demonstrated the selected skill, the facilitator may place the nurses in groups of five to practise the skill. They can take on the following roles; patient, nurse, patient observer, nurse observer, and group coordinator. Each must move through each of the roles, and sufficient time must be set aside after each piece of role play for discussion of the performances. This feedback is most important; it is at this point that self-insights can be sharpened and good techniques reinforced. However, unless such discussions are carefully controlled they can harm individuals. Undue criticism or embarrassment will discourage sensitive nurses.

The group facilitator must guide such discussions so that they inform, build up confidence and promote openness and peer support. Nurses can learn to support each other, and this is invaluable in the clinical situation. The nurse must be made aware that she is not expected to solve a patient's problems; only help him accept responsibility for solving his own problems. Finally, she should be taught the value of referral. Frequently she will be best able to help a patient by referring him to someone whose training, experience or availability will be of special assistance; for example, a ward sister, social worker, or hospital chaplain. Referral must never be interpreted as incompetence, and it should be done in such a way that the patient does not feel dismissed. Nurses need the maturity to accept and respond openly to the needs of students and those with less experience than themselves who are still struggling to develop a coherent self-image. Secure in your own self-image, you should remain open to continual learning. Your personal view of the world is one among many; and your ethical standards, whatever their intrinsic merit, may not be shared by a new generation of nurses. Moralising has no place in counselling or in the teaching of counselling. Nurses will become competent counsellors through developing self-awareness, and related experiences of helping patients to cope with their problems. You, as an experienced professional will be their sounding board and companion along the way.

References
Burton, G. (1979) Interpersonal Relations. Tavistock publications, London.
Collins, G. (1985) Christian Counselling. Hazell Watson and Viney Ltd, Aylesbury.
Heasman, K. (1969) Introduction to Pastoral Counselling. Constable, London.
Hurding, R.F. (1980) Restoring the Image. Paternoster Press, Exeter.
Minshill, D. (1982) Counselling in psychiatric nursing. *Nursing Times*, 7 July.
Rogers, C. (1961), On Becoming a Person. Constable, London.
Salaman, G. (1983) Counselling organisations: trust or conspiracy? *Nursing Times*, 19 January.
Spy, T. and Stone, J. (1982) So you think you know about counselling? *Nursing Times*, 21 May.
Stewart, W. (1979) Health Service Counselling. Pitman Medical Publishing Co., London.
Tournier, P. (1957) The Meaning of Persons. SCM Press Ltd., London.
Tschudin, V. (1982) Counselling Skills for Nurses. Balliere Tindall, London.
Wallis, J.H. (1973) Personal Counselling. Allen and Unwin, London.

11

Counselling: basic principles in nursing

Philip Burnard, MSc, RGN, RMN, DipN, CertEd, RNT
Lecturer in Nursing, Department of Nursing Studies, University of Wales, Cardiff

During the past five years the idea that nurses in all specialties should develop appropriate skills in communicating with and helping their patients has received much attention. Often, however, basic counselling skills are taught without supporting theoretical rationale. This chapter sets out some basic principles based on those found in humanistic psychology theory and in the literature on client-centred therapy, with the aim of offering a 'theoretical scaffolding' on which to build good practice. The principles are presented dogmatically for the sake of clarity but, like all principles, they are open to debate, clarification and development. A further reading list is offered to be used as a guide to tracing the ideas back to source.

The terms 'counsellor' and 'client' are used through the chapter. 'Counsellor' means any grade of nurse acting as counsellor. 'Client' means anyone with whom the nurse is interacting in a counselling capacity. Thus a client may be a patient, a colleague or a friend. Table 1 shows the basic principles of counselling.

1. The client knows best what is best for them.
2. Interpretation by the counsellor is likely to be inaccurate and is best avoided.
3. Advice is rarely helpful.
4. The client occupies a different 'personal world' from that of the counsellor and vice versa.
5. Listening is the basis of the counselling relationship.
6. Counselling 'techniques' should not be overused; however:
7. Counselling can be *learned*.

Table 1. Basic principles in counselling.

The client knows what is best for them   We all perceive the world differently having had different personal histories which colour our views. Throughout our lives we develop a variety of coping strategies and problem solving abilities which we use when beset by personal problems. Central to client-centred counselling is the idea that, given the space and time, we are the best arbiters of what is and is not right for us. We can listen to others, and hear their ideas but in the end we as individuals have to decide upon our own course of action.

Belief in the essential ability of all people to make worthwhile decisions for themselves arises from the philosophical tradition of existentialism. Existentialism argues, among other things, that we are born free and that we 'create' ourselves as we go through life. For the existentialist, nothing is predetermined, there is no blueprint for how any given person's life will turn out. Responsibility and choice lie squarely with the individual.

No one is free in all respects. We are born into a particular society, culture, family and body. On the other hand, our *psychological* make up is much more fluid and arguably not predetermined. We are free to think and feel. One of the *aims* of counselling is to enable the client to realise this freedom to think and feel.

Once a person has to some extent, recognised this freedom, he begins to realise that he can change his life. Again, in humanistic or client-centred counselling, this is a central issue: that people can change. They do not have to be weighed down by their past or by their conditioning (as psychoanalytical and behavioural theory would argue): they are more or less free to choose their own future. And no one can choose that future for them. Hence the overriding principle that the client knows what is best for them.

Interpretation by the counsellor is likely to be inaccurate and is best avoided To interpret, in this sense, is to offer the client an explanation of his thinking, acting or feeling. Interpretations are useful in that they can help to clarify and offer a theoretical framework on which the client may make future decisions. However, they are best left to the client to make.

As we have seen, we all live in different perceptual worlds. Because of this, another person's interpretation of *my* thinking, acting or feeling will be based on that person's experience — not mine. That interpretation is, therefore, more pertinent to the person offering it than it is to me, coloured as it is bound to be by the perceptions of the other person. Such colouring is usually more of a hindrance to me than a help.

It is tempting for others to lace their interpretations of a person's action with 'oughts' or 'shoulds'. Thus an interpretation can quickly degenerate into moralistic advice which may lead to the client feeling guilty or rejecting the advice because it does not fit into his own belief or value system.

Advice is rarely helpful Any attempt to help to 'put people's lives right' is fraught with pitfalls. Advice is rarely directly asked for and rarely appropriate. If it is taken, the client tends to assume that 'that's the course of action I would have taken anyway' or, he becomes dependent on the counsellor. The counsellor who offers a lot of advice is asking for the client to become dependent. Eventually, of course, some of the advice turns out to be wrong and the spell is broken: the counsellor is seen to be 'only human' and no longer the necessary life-line perceived by the client in the past. Disenchantment quickly follows and the client/counsellor relationship tends to degenerate rapidly. It is better then, not to become an advice-giver in the first place.

There are exceptions to this principle where advice giving is appropriate; about wound care or medication for example. In the sphere of personal problems, however, advice-giving is rarely appropriate.

Different 'personal worlds' of client and counsellor Because of varied experiences, different physiologies and shifting belief and value systems, we perceive the world through different 'frames of reference'. We act according to our particular belief about how the world is. What happens next, however, is dependent upon how the world *really* is. If there is a considerable gap between our 'personal theory of the world' and 'how the world really is' we may be disappointed or shocked by the outcome of our actions.

It is important that the counsellor realises that her own belief system may not be shared by the client and that her picture of the world is not necessarily more accurate.

A useful starting point is for the counsellor to explore her own belief and value system before she starts. She may be surprised at the contradictions and inconsistencies that abound in that 'personal world'! She is then in a better position to appreciate the difference between her belief system and her client's.

The counsellor's task is to attempt to enter and share the personal world of the client. This is often described as developing empathy or the ability to non-judgementally understand the particular view of the world that a person has at a particular time. That view usually changes as counselling progresses, after which the client may no longer feel the need for the counsellor. When this happens, the counsellor must develop her own strategies for coping with the separation that usually follows.

Counselling is a two-way process. While the client's personal world usually changes, so may the counsellor's. It can, then, be an opportunity for growth for the counsellor as well as the client.

Listening is the basis of the counselling relationship To really listen to another person is the most caring act of all, and takes skill and practice. Often, when we claim to be listening we are busy rehearsing our next verbal response, losing attention and failing to hear the other person. Listening involves giving ourselves up completely to the other person in order to fully understand.

We cannot listen properly if we are constantly judging or categorising what we hear. We must learn to set aside our own beliefs and values and to 'suspend judgement'. It is a process of offering free attention; of accepting, totally, the other person's story, accepting that their version of how the world is may be as valid as our own. Listening can be developed through practice and may be enhanced through meditation. Various experiential exercises have been developed to enable people to learn properly. They need to be used carefully with plenty of time allocated for them.

We need to listen to the metaphors, the descriptions, the value judgements and the words that people use, as they are all indicators of their personal world. Noting facial expressions, body movements, eye contact or lack of it, are all aspects of the listening process.

Many of us have been confronted by the neophyte counsellor whose determined eye-contact and stilted questioning make us feel distinctly uncomfortable! The aim is to gradually incorporate techniques into the personal repertoire. It is important that learner nurses do not adopt, wholesale, a collection of techniques that they have been taught in the school of nursing.

Counselling 'techniques' should not be overused If we arm ourselves with a whole battery of counselling techniques, perhaps learned through workshops and courses, we are likely to run into problems. The counsellor who uses too many techniques may be perceived by the client as artificial, cold and even uncaring. It is possible to pay so much attention to techniques that they impede listening and communicating.

Some techniques, such as the conscious use of questions, reflections, summary, probing and so forth are very valuable. What one must hope for, is that through practice, such techniques become natural to the counsellor. The process takes considerable time and must be rooted in a conscious effort to appear natural and spontaneous to others.

Counselling can be learned Counselling is not something that comes naturally to some and not to others. We can all develop listening skills and our ability to communicate clearly with other people, which is the basis of counselling. The skills can only be learned through personal experience and lots of practice, which may be gained in experiential learning workshops for development of counselling skills.

The list of principles outlined here is not claimed to be exhaustive. It attempts to identify *some* of the important principles involved and to explain them. The next stage is to develop counselling theory and skill further through reading and counselling skills courses. The bibliography identifies some sources of further ideas regarding the theory of counselling. These are not the *only* books on counselling but they are up-to-date, readable and currently available in bookshops.

Counselling skills courses are run by a variety of university extra-mural departments; by specialist counselling organisations and, increasingly, as part of the continuing education programmes organised with schools of nursing.

Bibliography

Bond, M. (1986) Stress and Self Awareness: A Guide for Nurses. Heinemann, London.
  A practical book which explores methods of coping with emotions and personal problems.

Burnard, P. (1985) Learning Human Skill: A Guide for Nurses. Heinemann, London.
  An introductory text on self-awareness and experiential learning. Contains a series of exercises on counselling skills training.

Burnard, P.(1989) Counselling Skills for Health Professionals. Chapman and Hall, London.
  A guide to many aspects of counselling theory and skills.

Claxton, G. (1984) Live and Learn: An Introduction to the Psychology of Growth and Change in Everyday Life. Harper and Row, London.
  A stimulating and eclectic approach to the question of how people learn and change. A very readable book.

Nelson-Jones, R. (1981) The Theory and Practice of Counselling Psychology. Holt, Rinehart Winston, London.
  A very comprehensive account of most aspects of counselling.

Rogers, C.R. (1980) A Way of Being. Houghton Mifflin, New York.
  A sensitive book by the late Carl Rogers founder of 'client-centred' counselling, which explores the nature of empathy and the therapeutic relationship.

12

Coping with other people's emotions

Philip Burnard MSc, RGN, RMN, DipN, CertEd, RNT
Lecturer in Nursing Studies, University of Wales College of Medicine, Cardiff

Nurses in all specialties regularly come into contact with people who are upset. In the psychiatric hospital, they are frequently asked to cope with those who are distressed as a result of depression, anxiety or fear. In the general hospital they also face the emotional release of others: in the intensive care unit, in medical, surgical and children's wards and also when relatives are distressed for any number of reasons. While there is an increasing focus on interpersonal and communication skills in all the nursing syllabi, the question of what to do when someone expresses strong emotion is still rarely addressed in a practical manner. This chapter outlines some of the options available to the nurse and suggests some guidelines for further training.

A healthy activity

The first consideration is that the release of emotion generally seems to be a *healthy* activity. We all have the capacity to express strong emotion (laughter, tears, anger and fear) and the release of such feeling tends to enable us to regain a certain equilibrium. Conversely, when we bottle up emotion we tend to function less effectively and often feel less healthy. Unfortunately, a cultural norm in this society seems to be that we should not outwardly show strong emotion: that we should maintain the 'stiff upper lip'. As a result, many people in our culture carry around with them a lot of unexpressed emotion. This can manifest itself in a variety of ways.

Physical tension A person carrying around a great deal of unexpressed anger, for example, will often experience considerable tension in the shoulders and upper trunk. One who cannot cope with their own unexpressed sorrow will ofter experience tension in their stomach. The mapping out of the physical effects of this emotional bottling up has been described by Reich (1976), who argues that release of such repressed emotion can lead to the person feeling more physically, as well as emotionally, stable and secure.

Emotional problems Emotional release often leads to the resolution of emotional problems. Thus the person who is grieving and allowed to express their grief will more readily come to terms with the loss they have experienced. It seems that the free expression of emotion is one of the means by which we come to terms with our problems. Again, the cultural norm runs counter to this principle and as a result many people think that it is not acceptable to express feeling openly. Such a sanction on the expression of feeling extends to nurses who often feel incompetent to deal with other people's emotional release.

Emotional release is a healthy process which can help people both physically and psychologically. The first way to help others in this area is to *allow* them to express feelings. If a relative or patient starts to cry, it is usually helpful to let them continue. For many nurses, the ingrained reflex when someone cries is to rush in and 'reassure' them in a rather desperate attempt to stop them crying. If we can resist that reflex and allow them to cry we will usually be helping them far more than if we offer them glib reassurance.

Such reassurance is often more for the nurse than for the patient. It is almost as if the patient's tears stir up our own unexpressed emotion and make us unhappy. As a result, we feel compelled to stop them. In the first place stopping them saves us the embarassment of not being able to deal with the emotion and in the second, it stops our own feelings from being churned up. If we, as nurses, are to deal with the emotional release of others frequently, we must take some time to consider our *own* emotional status. If we carry around a great deal of unexpressed emotion, we cannot expect to be much help to others when they are distressed. If our emotion is just beneath the surface, we will tend to avoid allowing others to freely release their feelings because we will find it too distressing.

Exploring our emotions

The first practical issue in helping others to express emotion, then, is to explore our own emotions. This can be done in a variety of ways. A support group can be set up to enable nurses to talk through their feelings about their job and, if necessary, their personal lives. Such groups can help relieve job-related stress and do much to ward off the development of burnout – the insidious process of exhaustion caused by job-related pressure. These groups can be set up by nurses who have had some experience and training in running groups, and training is regularly available in short workshops as part of extramural programmes of universities and colleges.

Support groups should meet once a week for an hour to be most effective. Any discussions which take place within them are confidential to group members. A useful book on running such groups is Ernst and Goodison's In Your Own Hands: a book of self-help therapy (1981), which gives details of how to set up, run and overcome teething troubles in support groups.

Individual nurses can make a contract with themselves to set aside time each day or week to talk through problems with a friend or trusted colleague. This may sound very formal, but unless we consciously set aside time to do this, the tendency is to allow ourselves to 'carry on as normal'. The net result is often that we do not communicate our feelings to others but continue to bottle them up. The process of setting aside time each week, in a fairly formal way, to talk things through can be very therapeutic. This can be shared equally between the two people involved and soon becomes a regular and very healthy part of the week.

Growth groups

A third approach to exploring personal feelings is to join a regular 'growth' group of some sort. Various types of women's and men's groups are now running up and down the country and they can be useful vehicles for the development of self-awareness and personal development. To some, the time taken up by such activities may seem self-indulgent, but if we are to truly help others, we must first help ourselves. Apart from the single sex groups mentioned here, there is a wide range of short courses and ongoing groups available through universities and colleges which aim to enhance self-awareness and develop communication skills. Co-counselling also offers a useful medium for exploring self development among trusted colleagues and friends. After initial training, co-counsellors meet regularly in pairs. One of the partners spends an hour in the role of 'client' and the other in that of 'counsellor', then the roles are reversed. The hour may be spent as the 'client' chooses: exploring problems, releasing pent-up emotion or planning for the future. Further details of co-counselling and co-counselling networks are described by Heron (1978).

Allowing the expression of emotion

This self-development is the first stage in preparing for helping others to express their emotions. The next stage is what to do when a person begins to express feelings, whether through tears, anger, fear or laughter. This expression is healthy, so the first 'rule' is to *allow* the expression of emotion. We have to learn to refrain from rushing to reassure the other person and from suggesting that they stop! If someone is 'allowed' to cry or express anger, the emotion usually runs its own course and they feel better as a result. If we rush in too quickly to stop the emotion, we encourage them to bottle things up and create potential problems for themselves later.

All we have to do, then, is to sit and allow the other person to release their feelings. This is easy to write about but often very difficult to do! We are nearly all readily programmed by our socialisation to jump in quickly to stop tears or anger. To sit back and 'allow' it is far more difficult. With conscious effort, backed up by exploration of our own emotional status, such acceptance can become our norm.

Nurses who regularly have to cope with profound emotional release are well advised to consider further training in cathartic methods. Issues such as when to intervene, when to encourage the release of emotion and *how* to encourage such release, need to be considered. Heron (1986) discusses many of these issues and his description of cathartic methods, their use and abuse makes useful reading. Cathartic work usually involves rather lengthy periods of time with the patient, and many nurses may feel that such an investment of time is an expensive one, but we are committed to caring for the *whole* person, then caring for their emotional needs is a high priority.

Therapeutic touch
One simple skill that all nurses have literally at their fingertips is the use of touch. Light touch can often promote and encourage emotional release, while an arm round the patient's shoulder is often comforting and interrupt their emotional release (Heron, 1986; Montague, 1978).

The third aspect of coping with other people's emotion is to allow a period after the tears or anger for them to 'make sense' of what has happened. This quiet period after the emotion has died down is an important aspect of the whole process. After expressing strong feeling, people are often flooded with new insights into their condition. It is as if the expression of feeling has allowed a veil to be lifted and that they now see things more clearly. Usually during this period, nothing need be said by the nurse at all. The patient (or relative) only needs to sit quietly and think things through. The insight that occurs during this period is often personal and it may not be expressed to the nurse. What is perhaps more important to the other person at this time is that they have *company* and are *allowed* the time they need to think things through in this way.

These, then, are three practical aspects of coping with other people's emotional release. First we explore our own emotions so that they do not 'get in the way' when the other person expresses feeling; second, we 'allow' full expression of the feeling, and third we allow time and space for the piecing together of the insights that usually follow such emotional release.

Emotional release is only part of a wide spectrum of interpersonal skills the nurse requires to satisfy patients' emotional needs. Heron (1986) offers a comprehensive and practical list of all possible types of therapeutic interventions which he calls Six Category Intervention Analysis (Heron, 1986). The therapeutic interventions that Heron identifies are as follows:

Prescriptive: the nurse offers suggestions or advice.

Informative: the nurse offers the patient factual information.

Confronting: the nurse challenges the patient.

Cathartic: the nurse helps the patient release pent-up emotion.

Catalytic: the nurse helps the patient to further consider their own thoughts and feelings by asking questions and generally 'drawing out' the patient.

Supportive: the nurse validates and encourages the patient.

Heron argues that the skilled practitioner can use all of these interventions appropriately. He also identifies non-therapeutic use of them and explains how each type of intervention can be misused. The nurse who develops skills in each of the six categories can become an effective helper in a range of interpersonal situations, with patients and their relatives and with her colleagues and friends. Once again, a variety of training courses in Six Category Intervention Analysis are available through various university departments and practical methods in the six categories are described elsewhere (Burnard, 1985).

It is interesting to note that recent research has suggested that trained nurses see themselves as skilled in using the prescriptive, informative and supportive categories but far less skilled in using the catalytic, confronting and cathartic categories (Burnard and Morrison, 1987).

The principles described in this article apply in almost all nursing settings: in clinical and community situations as well as in management and educational environments. All nurses can learn the basic skills involved in helping those who are emotionally distressed and so practise more therapeutically.

Increasingly, schools of nursing are using a range of experiential learning methods to facilitate the development of a wide range of interpersonal skills, such as counselling and group leadership. Perhaps more time needs to be set aside for the development of the specific skills of helping people to release emotion. Given the stressful nature of nursing, such competence can only help both nurse and patient. Perhaps, too, gradually and slowly, the cultural norm of keeping a stiff upper lip will change and a more completely human person will emerge.

References

Burnard, P. (1985) Learning Human Skills: A Guide for Nurses. Heinemann, London.

Burnard, P. and Morrison, P. (1987) Nurses' perceptions of their interpersonal skills. *Nursing Times*, 83, 42, 59.

Ernst, S. and Goodison, L. (1981) In Our own Hands: a book of self-help therapy. The Woman's Press, London.

Heron, J. (1978) Co-Counsellor's Teachers Manual. Human Potential Research Project, University of Surrey, Guildford.

Heron, J. (1986) Six Category Intervention Analysis (2nd Ed). Human Potential Research Project, University of Surrey, Guildford.

Montague, A. (1978) Touching: The Human Significance of the Skin. Harper and Row, New York.

Reich, W. (1976) Character Analysis. Simon and Schuster, New York.

Loss and
Bereavement

13

Helping clients to come to terms with loss

Teresa Lombardi, RGN, RSCN, RNT, Cert Ed, Dip Counselling
Senior Nurse Manager, Continuing Education, Worthing District School of Nursing

Working with terminally ill people, although rewarding and challenging, is far from easy, for a variety of reasons. It is impossible to identify a 'right and wrong' way of communicating with them, as each client has individual needs and ways of expressing him or herself. Similarly, each situation is different, and as nurses we bring our own individual attitudes, values, beliefs, experiences and skills into them. We also bring our feelings of anxiety and helplessness and our need to 'make it better' for patients or clients, which it is not always possible to do.

Witnessing strong emotions in others and learning to cope with and accept them may remind us of our own areas of difficulty and losses, whether real or feared. This can make us vulnerable to feelings of anxiety, inadequacy and pain. If we are not sufficiently aware of our own values, beliefs and areas of 'unfinished business', it may affect the way we relate to our clients and hinder the development of the qualities of warmth, acceptance, genuineness, empathy and flexibility that are so essential when working with this client group. Finally difficulties arise because ultimately 'effective helping' requires a degree of self confidence and courage and it is often easier to 'opt out' and avoid the situation. This is a normal coping strategy that we all need to do when we are vulnerable. We must care for ourselves as nurses or we will not be free to effectively care for others.

Tasks of mourning

Although each client and situation is different, there are certain principles that can be followed to make our helping skills more effective. It may be useful to consider these within the framework of the four tasks of mourning (Worden, 1983).

When clients are informed of their situation they often feel a sense of disbelief, that 'it is not really happening'. During this first stage the nurse's prime aim is to help the client become aware and accept that the situation is real, it is happening and is not a figment of the imagination. This is essential, as only when reality is accepted can the client progress and experience the pain of grief, ultimately moving through to resolution. One of the best ways to help clients accept their loss is to encourage them to talk. Many clients mentally relive where they were when they first heard of their diagnosis, what happened and who said what. They may need to talk through this again and again, over weeks or even months. While family and friends may grow tired and even impatient the effective nurse is a patient listener who encourages the clients to talk.

Acknowledging grief

The second task of mourning is to acknowledge and experience the pain of grief. Feelings such as anger, guilt and sadness may not be acceptable to either family or friends or to clients themselves. They may therefore try to suppress or even deny their pain in order to avoid burdening, distressing or embarrassing their loved ones, while other clients may think they are 'going mad'. During this stage clients need to be helped to give themselves 'permission' to be angry or sad, or to cry, and must be given opportunity to talk through their guilt and unburden themselves. A nurse's quiet acceptance and acknowledgement of the pain of grief will facilitate this difficult task, which means that clients are not left to carry the burden of their pain with them into the next stage of their lives.

Adjustment

The third task of mourning is that of adjusting to the loss, real or impending. Essentially the nurse helps clients to identify problems and then to explore alternative ways of dealing with them. For example, this may mean identifying short term goals, of looking at today and next week rather than next month or next year. This is an active stage and may involve adopting and coming to terms with a new role or learning new skills such as coping with a prosthesis.

The final stage of mourning involves withdrawing emotional energy from the loss and reinvesting it in another relationship or diverting it to other channels. At this point the intense pain of grief diminishes and although clients will still experience a sense of sadness they will be able to channel their emotions into living and dealing with their lives today.

Skills for effective helping

Effective helping can be viewed as a problem solving activity. Most nurses use a variety of skills throughout the helping process and although there is no standard classification of such skills, for convenience they can be divided into two main stages.

Stage one — attending Effective helpers are those who can establish a caring, non threatening relationship with their clients. Many nurses begin this relationship with an advantage in that the client's trust is already invested in them because of the nurturing nature of the nursing role. Trust will also develop if the nurse can be open and honest — relationships bound by any degree of mutual pretence will lead to feelings of insecurity and non-acceptance in clients (Glaser and Strauss, 1965), who will then be more likely to withdraw into their lonely worlds.

The first contact between nurse and client is crucial in developing and maintaining a warm trusting relationship. The client will have doubts and fears, and some problems will seem too large, too overwhelming or too unique to share. He may ask himself, ''Can I really trust this person?'', ''Is she really interested in me?'' ''Does she have the time for me?'' Answers to such questions will be provided not merely by words but by other more subtle and powerful means of communication. The physical setting, the way the nurse greets the client and her gestures and tone of voice can all convey sensitivity and consideration.

Observing and reacting

From the first meeting nurse and client will engage in the process of observing and reacting to the other. Success in helping depends upon the client's perception of the nurse's manner and behaviour. He will look for, and must experience, empathy, respect and sensitivity. Being with, attending to and listening are supportive and comforting behaviours which convey respect and concern for the client.

At this stage an opening statement such as, ''I wonder what worries you have about your illness?'' may provide the necessary invitation for the client to take the lead and talk freely while the nurse 'attends'. This involves 'being with' the client physically and psychologically. Body communication, posture, degree of relaxation and eye contact indicate interest in and attention to the client. Attending behaviour encourages the trust that is so necessary for promoting exploration and will also help the nurse listen more effectively.

Listening is an active, complex process and perhaps the most important of all helping skills. It involves first observing and interpreting the client's non-verbal behaviour and then listening to and interpreting his verbal messages. During the process of listening, the skill of reflection can be used by the nurse to sensitively communicate to the client her understanding of his concerns. It is an empathetic response that involves restating in fresh words the client's core feelings. For example:

Client: ''I'm bewildered, there's so much to take in and consider, and so many different doctors each with their own ideas.''

Nurse: ''It all seems so confusing, even overwhelming and almost out of your control.''

Client: ''Yes, that's it, it feels like that.''

An accurate reflection, while not halting the flow of talk can help clarify and bring less obvious feelings into the client's awareness so that they can be 'owned' and acknowledged. Reflection also increases the degree of trust which will ultimately facilitate further exploration.

Stage two — responding This stage of helping involves maintaining the good relationship developed in the first stage and taking the process further by helping the client explore, clarify and define his problem or area of concern. Responding skills help the client progress through the stages of mourning, the appropriate and effective ones at this stage are those which enable the client to extend and develop his understanding of himself and his difficulties.

Effective helping will be determined by the nurse's ability to respond accurately to the needs and cues provided by the client. This 'staying with the client' demonstrates empathy and acceptance. To achieve this the nurse needs to avoid directing and leading, eg "I don't think you should be spending so much time talking about your illness."; reassuring, eg "That's a common problem, but you'll be alright."; advising, eg "I wouldn't tell your family about this;" or not accepting the client's feelings and hiding behind the professional facade, eg "Your depression will pass, it's just part of the body's response to your treatment."

Staying with the client may also mean staying silent if he needs time to gather thoughts and feelings together. Although there are many different meanings for a silence, it is often a productive time and it is helpful if the nurse simply waits quietly until the client is ready to go on. This is perhaps a very difficult strategy to adopt as we are used to commenting on, advising or teaching.

Other skills

Other responding skills which will help exploration and clarification are probing, questioning and summarising. Prompts and probes are verbal tactics which help clients talk about themselves and define their problems more concretely. A prompt may be a head nod or a simple "Aha" or "I see" while a probe may take the form of a statement, eg "When you were told you had cancer you said you were both relieved and depressed. I'm wondering how you've been since then."

The careful use of questions can also help focus and clarify. These should be open questions, usually beginning with 'how', 'what' or 'who', which leave the respondent free to answer as he wishes, eg "Can you explain what you mean?", or "What was it about your treatment session today that was so upsetting?". Asking too many questions, however, may make the client feel interrogated, anxious and insecure, which will interfere with the rapport between nurse and client. Questions which begin with 'why', such as, "Why did you feel like that?" are also unhelpful, as they lead the client to search for intellectual explanations to justify his feelings.

Summarising

Summarising is the process of tying together all that has been communicated during part or all of a helping session. It can also be a natural means of finishing the session or beginning a new one. This then paves the way for the client to commit himself to further exploration and to developing awareness. Thus, with continuing emotional support the client, finding and utilising his own inner resources, moves on with hope to another day.

These strategies have been identified to help the nurse care for clients who are experiencing loss, but it should be remembered that the nurse has to deal with her own personal feelings of grief in response to the client's situation. In addition she may be constrained by fears that she will make the situation worse for the client through lack of skill. Only the client can judge what is helpful and is likely to seek a nurse who can support, comfort and care, and is herself — a real person with strengths and weaknesses like anyone else.

Bibliography
Brammer, L. M. (1979) The Helping Relationship Process and Skills. Prentice-Hall, New Jersey.
   Provides more in-depth discussion of the issues raised in this paper.
Egan, G. (1982) The Skilled Helper Model, Skills and Methods for Effective Helping. Brooks Cole Publishing Company, California.
   Describes in detail the skills and methods needed for effective helping.
Munro, E. A., Nanthei, R. J., Small, J.J. (1983) Counselling: A Skills Approach. Methuen, New Zealand.
   A clearly-written text with some very practical exercises and examples of helping skills.
Nelson-Jones, R. (1983) Practical Counselling Skills. Holt, Rinehart and Winston, London.
   Applies the theory of counselling in a very practical way using exercises to aid skill development and case studies as examples.

References
Glaser, B. and Strauss, A. (1965) Awareness of Dying. Aldine, Chicago.
Worden, W.J. (1983) Grief Counselling and Grief Therapy. Tavistock Publications, London.

14

Bereavement: the needs of the patient's family

Jenny Penson, MA, SRN, HVCert, Cert Ed, RNT
Senior Lecturer in Nursing Studies, Dorset Insitute of Higher Education

Through this chapter bereaved people are referred to as "family" or "relatives" for ease of comprehension. Terms such as "key people" or "significant others", while rather unwieldy, may more accurately describe the grieving person who is, for example, a life-long friend.

"Bereavement" means "to be robbed of something valued" – this definition seems particularly helpful as it indicates that this someone or something has been wrongly or forcibly taken from you. A key concept to understanding bereavement is that of loss. As Caplan (1964) and others have suggested, the grief experienced after losing someone close to you may be similar to the emotions felt after other types of loss, life transitions such as redundancy, divorce, failing an important exam or losing a much loved pet. As nurses we become aware of the emotions that patients experience after operations such as mastectomy, amputation of a limb or the loss of body image caused by suffering from a disfiguring disease.

When people are bereaved they suffer not only the loss of a person but also a substantial part of themselves, because everything they have shared with that person cannot be repeated with anyone else. The bereavement experience, therefore, is one of strong, violent and sometimes overwhelming reactions. These feelings actually begin from the moment the relative is told that the patient will not recover, referred to by Lindemann (1944) as "anticipatory grief".

The patient

Kubler Ross (1970), states: "We cannot help the terminally ill patient in a really meaningful way if we do not include his family." She determined that family members undergo stages of adjustment similar to the five phases she described for dying patients – denial, anger, bargaining, depression and acceptance as they come to terms with the reality of terminal illness in the family. She advocates that when there is time to do so, the family should be encouraged to express grief as much as possible prior to the death of a loved one which serves to alleviate, to some extent, the pain that is felt afterwards. If members of a family can share these emotions they will gradually face the reality of the impending separation and come to an acceptance of it together.

Unresolved family stress can significantly affect the outcome of the patient's illness, so the care of the family is part of the total care of the patient. It is also about understanding him as a member of the family group, and being aware that he and his family are not separate entities. Each constantly influences the other, thus affecting the health and happiness of both. It is possible that nursing actions may affect the long-term adjustment of the bereaved relatives after the death of the patient.

Molter (1979) studied family needs as they identified them, and looked at whether these were being met, and if so, by whom. The results showed that relatives could identify their needs during an intensive phase of hospitalisation. Their universal and strongest need was for hope. Nurses can go some way towards meeting this need by helping to set short-term goals for the patient. A weekend at home, a visit from a favourite friend, planning something special to enjoy together all helps to relieve that sense of helplessness which is often felt. They also go some way towards providing good memories to look back on. Reassurance that the patient will not be allowed to suffer pain or great distress, that someone will be with them when they die, and that support is available after the death if they need it, are all significant to those for whom no hope of an ultimate recovery can be given.

Hampe (1975) also found that spouses believed that the nurse's primary responsibility was to the patient and therefore they would be too busy to help relatives. One of the principal needs she identified from her study was for the family to be able to visit the dying patient at any time and for as long as they wished. They also wanted prompt help with the physical care and a demonstration of friendliness and concern in their relationship with the nurse.

My own experience indicates that encouraging involvement of the family in the care of the patient may minimise feelings of guilt during bereavement. There is a sense of not having failed when one was needed and the satisfaction of having done something tangible to give comfort and show love.

Hospital or home care?
This must be borne in mind when discussing the pros and cons of hospital versus home care. Where dying at home is possible because both the patient and their relatives want it, and there are enough resources available when needed, the family are likely to feel a sense of achievement, of not having failed the patient. On the other hand, relatives do derive comfort from the security of constant professional expertise and the knowledge that any emergency will be dealt with by a 24-hour service. However, they still need to feel involved and should

be encouraged to give to the patient in any way they can. This might range from helping with nursing care to arranging photos and flowers or bringing in special food or drink that the patient may ask for which the hospital cannot supply.

To tell or not to tell

Whether or not to tell the patient of his diagnosis and prognosis is a dilemma which causes much distress to family, patients and nurses. Sometimes relatives are advised by doctors and/or nurses not to be truthful with the patient and this can create a barrier between them, described by Solzhenitsyn (1971) as "a wall of silence" which separates them.

There is an obvious conflict in many relatives' minds between the idea of the patient's right to autonomy to knowing the truth if he wishes it, and the idea of paternalism, having the right to withhold it on the grounds of protecting the patient and giving him hope. Relatives will often say such things as "it will be too much for him", "he will give up", "I know he won't be able to stand it", "he will be frightened". These sort of statements may well be true but they may also reflect the relatives' own fears.

The cue to how much information is given should lie with the patient and the nurse's role with the relatives is often to explain to and sustain them during that gradual realisation that comes to most patients near the end. This may or may not be expressed and shared. However, when a patient and family can openly discuss their situation together, their relationship can be deepened and this can give great comfort to the bereaved person afterwards. It also creates a basis of honesty and trust which facilitates the relationship between patient, family and carers. Ann Oakley (1985) described when her father, Richard Titmuss, was dying: "You said things you never would have said had you not known you were dying – and that is how I knew you were."

That families fail to share their feelings openly with one another when faced with terminal illness may be due to the defence of denial and also a function of experience. Although we, the health workers, have been enlightened about combating this so-called conspiracy of silence which surrounds the topic of death, it is also possible that some families have been over-exposed to that viewpoint. As Bowen, (1978) points out, in spite of whatever attitudinal change that may have taken place the "basic problem is an emotional one and a change in the rules does not automatically change the emotional reactivity."

Support

So, should staff be so involved as to sit and weep with the relatives? Is this what sharing and support is about? Kubler Ross, (1974), suggests that we ask ourselves whether we would judge someone who cared enough to cry for us. "A display of emotions on the part of the therapist is like drugs, the right amount of medicine at the right time can work wonders. Too much is unhealthy – and too little is tragic."

It has been suggested that nurses are in a prime position to meet the family needs through active listening and supporting. They found that relatives wanted support but they tended to feel they should not burden the "too busy" nurses with their problems. It is important, therefore, that a sense of availability is conveyed to families so that they will not feel guilty when sharing fears and worries with the nurse. Families usually appreciate information and explanation about nursing procedures, tests, treatments, medications. This helps them to feel they are part of the life of the patient and increases feelings of control, which can enable them to cope more realistically and effectively with the immediate future.

Relatives who feel that they have not been "told enough" are suffering from a lack of sustained professional interest. Effective nursing care is *planned* care and relatives can and should be involved in this. Short-term objectives for the patient such as an improved night's sleep, can be explained to relatives and are positive indicators that there are always things which can be done to improve the quality of life for the patient.

There is often an accompanying aspiration or, for many people, a desperate need to find that the experience of grieving does have some meaning. This may lead to a turning or returning towards religion, or other philosophies of living. The nurse can often meet this need with tact and sensitivity by introducing the hospital chaplain or family priest at an appropriate moment. Their availability to families as well as patients gives comfort, and helps them to explore their own beliefs and what they mean.

Physical fitness is related to the ability to cope with stress and measures to maintain health may be more acceptable to the family if they are seen in terms of enabling them to support and be with the dying patient. They also serve to reinforce the message that the grieving relative *is* an important individual whose needs are also the nurse's concern. Simple relaxation techniques to promote sleep and encouragement to eat regularly are all part of this care.

Interpersonal skills

It is important, therefore, for nurses to develop interpersonal skills to enable them to meet the needs of the patient's family. The creation of a trusting relationship, the ability to give information in a clear and sympathetic manner, the ability to listen actively to their concerns and to help them to clarify problems and options all involve skills which can be learned and practised.

As Frederick and Frederick (1986) point out, although there is a great deal of controversy surrounding anticipatory grief, it appears that it may be a way of doing some of the work of mourning before the death occurs. In this way, it may soften the impact of the actual death on the bereaved.

The nurse is in a unique position, being in constant contact with the family. Her attention to their needs may have long-term beneficial effects on their adjustment to bereavement and is likely to enhance the quality of their remaining time with the dying patient.

References

Bowen, M. (1978) Family reactions to death. In: Family Therapy and Clinical Practice. Aronson, New York.

Caplan, G. (1964) Principles of Preventive Psychiatry. Basic Books, New York.

Frederick, J.F. and Frederick, N.J. (1985) The hospice experience: possible effects in altering the biochemistry of bereavement. *Hospice Journal*, **1**, 3, 81-89.

Hampe, S. (1975) Needs of the grieving spouse in a hospital setting. *Nursing Research*, **24**, 20.

Kubler-Ross, E. (1970) On Death and Dying. Tavistock, London.

Kubler-Ross, E. (1974) Questions and Answers on Death and Dying. Macmillan, London.

Lindemann, E. (1944) Symptomatology and management of acute grief. *American Journal of Psychiatry*, 101, 141-149.

Molter, N.C. (1979) Needs of critically ill patients: a descriptive study. *Nursing Research*, **8**, 2.

Oakley, A. (1985) Taking it Like a Woman. Penguin, London.

Solzhenitsyn, A. (1971) Cancer Ward. Penguin, London.

Ward, A.W.M. (1976) Mortality of bereavement. *British Medical Journal*, **11**, 700-102.

15

Terminal care: their death in your hands

Suzanne Conboy-Hill, PhD, MPhil, BA, SRN, AFBPsS
Principal Psychologist, Brighton Health Authority

There has recently been a dramatic increase in interest in the care of dying people and research into how this can be given. However, this appears to reflect rather than precede the growth of the hospice movement, and so understanding of the needs of dying people, their families, friends and carers remains scanty in hospitals, despite the fact that increasing numbers of people are being admitted to hospital for terminal care.

Recent improvement in research
This chapter is a short review of psychological and nursing literature in terminal care with some suggested changes nurses might make to ensure the maximum relief of psychological as well as physical pain in dying people.

Much of the research work in terminal care, initiated primarily by such people as Elizabeth Kubler-Ross and Cicely Saunders, has been carried out in America by groups comprising medics, nurses, theologians and psychologists (eg McCusker, 1984; Friel and Tehan, 1980; Davis and Jessen, 1981). While earlier work may be criticised for being largely made up of case histories or anecdotes, the more recent studies have been objective and systematic applications of the scientific method. Nurses in particular have become extremely skilled in this area.

Some interesting findings have been accumulated in these studies, many suggesting that health care personnel are surprisingly ill-prepared to deal with the psychological aspects of dying, so that many terminally ill people get rather a raw deal (Backer et al, 1982).

While most ordinary people would imagine that hospital work must inure its staff to the distress of facing dying people, enabling them to give the best possible care, research shows that both doctors and nurses consistently avoid social contact with terminal patients and that medical students learn early in their careers to become less available to them (eg Doka, 1982; LeShan, 1969; Rabin and Rabin, 1970; Todd and Still, 1984).

It is not clear why this should be, but research has shown that doctors themselves are more, rather than less, afraid of death (Schoenberg and Carr, 1972) and, being in executive control of patient care, frequently deny patients the right to know of their prognosis (Ley, 1977). This puts nurses in the invidious position of knowing the facts but being unable to discuss them with patients or relatives if they are asked.

Effects on nursing care

This may have several effects. Nurses may find ways of talking to dying people without giving any information — perhaps by offering reassurances or platitudes; they may experience conflict which leads to burnout and eventually leave the profession or they may develop patterns of care which avoid social behaviour with dying people. There is evidence for all of these. Nurses describe feelings of helplessness, inadequacy and depression associated with terminal care (Wilson, 1985; Friel and Tehan, 1980; Mandel, 1981). They often use subtle avoidance and conversation-controlling tactics while taking care of the physical needs of dying people (Nicholls, 1984). This poor communication means that people often remain ignorant of the details of their illness while almost everyone else has been given some, if not all, the relevant information.

If research had shown that dying people have no insight into their prognosis and that the distress is clearly confined to health care personnel themselves, then future research should be directed towards enabling staff to 'let sleeping dogs lie' in the most positive way. However, it would seem that patients do have insight into their condition and so are being denied the opportunity to discuss their prognosis and the emotional and practical consequences openly and honestly with those upon whom they would normally rely (Hinton, 1967; Todd and Still, 1984; Antonovsky, 1972).

Closed awareness

The distress associated with this situation, which is known as 'closed awareness', has been observed consistently by those working in the field (eg Hinton, 1967; Cassem and Stewart, 1975; Howells, 1983). Patients themselves have reported relief when open awareness is established (Kubler-Ross, 1969; see also Backer et al, 1982).

This evidence should not be seen as a prescription for routine or ruthless truth telling. Braver (1985) asks, 'Which patient, what truth?', implying a very individual approach is needed, and Hinton (1967) feels that simply telling people is the wrong approach because it suggests that the teller knows everything and the patient nothing. He recommends sensitive interview procedures which allow what Schoenberg and others have called 'graded honesty', and points out how important it is that interviewers be readily available to listen, so that they are always in touch with the patient's current needs.

Should nurses take control?

Nurses are clearly best placed for this role and Benoliel (1972) has gone as far as suggesting that nurses rather than doctors take executive control of care when it becomes predominantly comfort oriented rather than curative. Of course, with current emphasis on an inter-disciplinary team approach to care, it could be argued that no-one should take complete control. However, it is clear that this ideal has a long way to go and nurses may have to exert their authority in some particular way before gaining acceptance as true equals in a team containing medical practitioners.

To do this, nurses will need to:

● confront doctors about their joint role in information exchange, aiming to gain the right to independent practice in dealing with the day to day psychological needs of patients;

● generate research tied to patients' psychological needs and those of their carers (staff and families);

● develop training methods based on research and continuing through basic and post-basic education;

● develop and evaluate ways of stress management for staff working in terminal care (Mandel, 1981).

An authoritative, informed and assertive nursing staff, abandoning what has been described as the traditional doctor/nurse, male/female role model (Field, 1982), may be essential for the development of good psychosocial care of dying people. Only then can honest relationships develop, allowing patients to place trust and confidence in those to whom they must increasingly surrender control.

References

Antonovsky, A. (1972) The image of four diseases held by the urban Jewish population of Israel. *Journal of Chronic Disease.*

Backer, B. A., Hannon, N. and Russess, N.A. (1982) Death and Dying. Wiley & Son.

Benoliel, J. (1972) Nursing care for the terminal patient; a psychosocial approach. I Schoenberg et al, (Eds) Psychosocial Aspects of Terminal Care, 145.

Braver, P. (1965) Should the patient be told the truth? In Skipper, J. and Leonard, R. (Eds), Social Interaction and Patient Care. Lippincott, Philadelphia.

Cassem, N.H. and Stewart, R.S. (1975) Management and care of the dying patient. *International Journal of Psychiatry in Medicine,* 6, 1/2, 293.

Davies, G. and Jessen, A. (1981) An experiment in death education in the medical curriculum. *Omega J. Death and Dying,* 11, 2, 157.

Doka, K. (1982) The social organisation of terminal care in two paediatric hospitals. *Omega J. Death and Dying,* 12, 2, 129.

Field, D. (1983) Study of nurses engaged in terminal care on an acute medical ward. Paper presented to British Psychological Society Conference, York.

Friel, M. and Tehan, C.B. (1980) Counteracting burnout for the hospice caregiver. *Cancer Nursing,* Aug. 285.

Hinton, J. (1967) Dying. Pelican, London.

Howells, K. (1983) Teaching the medical profession about death and dying. Paper presented to British Psychological Society Conference, York.

Kubler-Ross, E. (1969) On Death and Dying. Macmillan, New York.

LeShan, L. (1969) Psychotherapy and the dying patient. In Pearson, L. (Ed), Death and Dying. The Press of Case Western University, Cleveland.

Ley, P. (1977) Psychological studies of doctor-patient communication. In Rackham, S. (Ed), Contributions to Medical Psychology. Pergamon Press.

McCusker, J. (1984) Development of scales to measure satisfaction and preferences regarding long-term and terminal care. *Medical Care,* 22, 5, 476.

Mandel, H. (1981). Nurses' feelings about working with the dying. *American Journal of Nursing,* 816, 1194.

Nicholls, K. (1984) Psychological Care in Physical Illness. Croom Helm.

Rabin, D. and Rabin, L. (1970) In Brim, O. et al (Eds), The Dying Patient. Russell Sage Foundation, New York.

Schoenberg, B. and Carr, A. (1972) Educating the health professional in the psychosocial care of the terminally ill. In Schoenberg, B., et al (Eds), Psychosocial Aspects of Terminal Care. Columbia University Press.

Todd, C.J. and Still, A.W. (1984) Communication between general practitioners and patients dying at home. *Soc.Sci.Med.* **18**, 8, 667.

Wilson, C. (1985) Stress in hospice nursing. *News Letter of the British Psychological Society Division of Clinical Psychology*, No 48, 5.

Teamwork

16

Teamwork: an equal partnership?

Gill Garrett, BA SRN, RCNT, DN(London), CertEd(FE), RNT, FPCert
Freelance Lecturer, Bristol

From being one of the fundamental tenets in the care of groups such as elderly people and those with mental handicaps, the vital nature of the team approach has become recognised and accepted in all areas of nursing. Many patients have a multiplicity of needs – medical, nursing, therapeutic, social – which no one discipline can hope to meet; only by close collaboration and cooperation can different practitioners bring their skills into concert to attempt to meet them.

Increasingly in recent years, the validity of this contention has been appreciated by both hospital and community workers, and the gospel has been preached. But how effective has the concept been in practice? While no doubt in many parts of the country teams are working efficiently and harmoniously together to the benefit of all concerned, it would seem that in others there are areas of concern which demand urgent consideration and action if the concept is not to prove a meaningless cliché. With this in mind, this chapter considers the prerequisites for effective teamwork, points out a few of the common problems which may arise and offers some suggestions as to how these problems may be ameliorated.

Who makes up the team?

One very basic question to ask before considering the work of the team is who makes up the team? On multiple choice papers, students will indicate the doctor, nurse, therapists, dietitians – all the professional partners in the venture. But integral to every team must be the people most meaningful to the individual patient: her family if she has any, her supportive neighbour, or whoever. If our aim is to rehabilitate the patient or to maintain her at her maximum level of functioning, these are people we neglect at our peril – and much more importantly, at the patient's peril. As professionals we must learn that we do not have a monopoly on care, nor do we have a dominant role in an unequal partnership. The contribution of relatives or friends, as agreeable to the patient, is vital – whether discussing assessments, setting goals or reviewing progress; their non-contribution, if excluded from active participation, may indeed frustrate all professional efforts. Although most of this article concentrates on those professionals who are conventionally seen as team members (primarily because of the space available), this point cannot be overstressed.

Why are teams necessary?

Perhaps an even more basic question is, why does the team exist? It is easy to lose sight of the fact that its sole *raison d'être* is the patient and her need. An old adage runs, "The patient is the centre of the medical universe around which all our works revolve, towards which all our efforts trend". In economic terms we are quite used to this concept of 'consumer sovereignty', but in our health and social services management at present, all too often our consumer exists more to be 'done to' rather than canvassed for her opinion, offered options and helped to make choices. A thorny question often raised about the multidisciplinary team is, which professional should lead it? An equally important one not so often posed is, who should be the 'director' of team activity? If we recognise the patient as an autonomous, independent person (albeit with varying degrees of support), surely we must have the humility to acknowledge that this directing role falls inevitably to her. For patients with mental or other serious impairment, of course, the question of advocacy then arises – again an issue subject to much current debate.

Having allocated the role of director to the patient, the team leader then becomes the facilitator of action. It has been said that, "Fundamental to the concept of teamwork is . . . division of labour, coordination and task sharing, each member making a different contribution, but (one) of equal value, towards the common goal of patient care" (Ross, 1986). What do these elements demand? To make for efficient division of labour there has to be an accurate assessment of a situation and the input needed to deal with it, a recognition of who is the best person for which part of the job, and the carrying through of the appropriate allocation. Coordination demands the ability to see the overall, the sum of all the individual parts, and to recognise their relative weightings in various circumstances; it needs effective communication skills and the ability to use feedback to take adjustive action as required. Task-sharing demands that team members have an understanding of different roles and their effect upon one another, that they recognise areas of overlap and are prepared to shoulder one another's problems should the need arise. Such demands are not light; they require considerable training and practice to perfect.

Status and power within the team

Consideration of the second part of the Ross quotation brings us to one of the common problems experienced in multidisciplinary teamwork: ". . . of equal value towards the common goal of patient care". Is that how all team members view their own contribution or that of their partners? Status and power imbalances can make for great difficulties in team functioning; tradition accords high status and consequent power to the medical establishment, for example, with much affection but little standing to nurses. But if nurses have been seen as lacking in power and status, even lower on the rungs of the ladder comes the patient; in general, society grants a very low status to ill and disabled people, and institutional care strips all vestiges of power from inhabitants.

For workers who see themselves as being the juniors in teams, the presence and influence of more powerful members may prove intimidating, and consequently they may make only tentative and limited contributions to discussions and meetings. It is important that they realise that, however 'junior', they have a right to contribute, indeed a duty to do so, if they have what has been described as the "authority of relevance" (Webb and Hobdell, 1975) – if they have knowledge relevant to the patient's own feelings of need or wellbeing which must be brought to the team's attention. So often it is those members who spend more time in close proximity to the patient who possess such authority, rather than the senior medical personnel who may visit her only on a weekly basis.

'Follow my leader'   A second problem may arise out of the power and status imbalance, especially when team members have become used to suppressing their views or do not recognise their authority of relevance – regression into the 'follow my leader' phenomenon. There may be the tendency to leave all the thinking to another group member who is perceived as being more prestigious or simply more articulate, often the consultant. His thinking and directions are seen as definitive, with team members abdicating their own professional responsibility to think and speak for themselves and for their patient from their own vantage points. Except in the unlikely event of the team leader being qualified in a multidisciplinary capacity, this obviously acts to the detriment of patient care – we can none of us prescribe or wholly substitute for each other's contributions. A variation on this 'follow my leader' phenomenon is sometimes seen where two leaders emerge from subgroups in a team, each with his or her own following. In addition to the drawbacks already mentioned, the results in situations like this are invariably divisive too.

'Groupthink'   This is the name that has been given to another possible problem in teamwork; it is generally seen in well-established, long-lived teams whose members over time have grown very used to working with each other. Team meetings are always amicable and 'cosy', there is no bickering or dissension and everyone gets on terribly well with everyone else. The group gives the appearance of having its own internal strength, with a marked sense of loyalty and supportiveness. But this denies that disagreement and conflict are facts of life and often signs of constructive enquiry and growth; all too often such teams ". . . become rigid, committed to the status quo . . . less open to input and feedback. Hierarchies become established and bureaucratic qualities emerge which resist questioning and change" (Brill, 1976).

Patient confusion   In case this should all seem a little esoteric, consider for a moment one last very basic possible problem in multidisciplinary teamwork – potential confusion for the patient. Unless each member of the team extends to her the courtesy of an introduction to their personal role, with an explanation of how this fits in with the overall individual plan of care, especially in the acute phase of an illness, the patient (particularly if elderly) may well find so many professionals overwhelming and muddling. If she is to feel in any degree in control of the situation and if any confusion is to be lessened, time must be taken to be sure a personal approach, with all care being presented as part of a concerted whole, and with common goals identified towards which all the team are working.

This last problem, then, is usually amenable to a common courtesy and common sense solution. But what about the others? The problems associated with status and 'follow my leader' have a more deep-seated origin and, although rectifiable in the short term in individual teams, in the longer term they demand a close scrutiny of, and changes in, professional education. 'Groupthink' demands flexibility of individuals and a system which encourages and permits a regular turnover of personnel to maintain healthy group dynamics.

Common core training?

If in effective teams there is no room for professional superiorities or jealousies, what is needed is an open, trusting relationship based on knowledge of, and respect for, one another's professional expertise. But this demands in turn an insight into other trainings and backgrounds to understand one another's terms of reference – the differences in emphasis we have in relation to patient care. While individual effort and inservice training programmes can go some way towards this, the difficulties with late attitudinal change are only too well known. Most of our basic feelings about our own profession and those with which we work are formed during our initial training period. Nursing is currently introducing training programmes based on Project 2000, with a common core foundation programme for all nurse practitioners. Is it not time we were much more adventurous, and explored avenues of common core training for all health professionals? Certain knowledge, skills and attitudes are prerequisites whether we are to be doctors, nurses, therapists or social workers – if we learned them together how much easier it would be to practise them together. The intention of such common training would not be to reduce all teaching to the lowest common denominator, but rather to look at areas of mutual concern, highlighting the unique contribution of each professional, and the bearing this has on the work of the other team members.

Value of difference

Educational change may also help us to recognise the value of 'difference' and the constructive use to which conflict may be put, so that 'groupthink' becomes a less likely problem. Better training in interpersonal skills – including assertiveness – should help the creation of a climate in which there is freedom to differ, to look more dispassionately at dissent, while acknowledging the areas of basic trust and agreement that do exist and can be built upon. The need for turnover in team membership has to be balanced, of course, by the need for reasonable stability over a period of time. Change every five minutes for the sake of it helps no one, but there must be recognition that long-term team stagnation (however well camouflaged) is beneficial neither to the group nor to the professionals within it – and certainly not to the patient and her family.

Realism

This chapter provides only a brief overview of a very important area. Readers' personal experiences may differ considerably from the scenarios which have been outlined. It would seem, however, that most experienced nurses have had the experience of needing to temper idealism in striving for effective teamwork with realism, given the situations in which they work. But recognition of this is in itself a step forward; we must have in mind that "under the aegis of teamwork, strange bedfellows are discovering, in time, that they must *learn* to work together before they *can* work together . . . teamwork is not an easy process to understand or to practise" (Brill, 1976).

References

Brill, N.I. (1976) Teamwork: Working together in the Human Services. Lippincott, New York.

Ross, F.M. (1986) Nursing old people in the community. In: Redfern, S. (ed) Nursing Elderly People. Churchill Livingstone, Edinburgh.

Webb, A.L. and Hobdell, M. (1975) Coordination between health and personal social services: a question of quality. In: Interaction of social welfare and health personnel in the delivery of services: Implications for training. Eurosound Report No. 4, Vienna.

17

Teamwork in psychiatry

Brendan McMahon, BA, SRN, RMN

Clinical Nurse Specialist in Dynamic Psychotherapy, Southern Derbyshire H.A.

Human beings have always needed each other. Medieval societies in Europe were based on the recognition that the peasant, the feudal lord, and the churchman was each necessary to the continued material and spiritual wellbeing of the community, and that the work performed by each was valuable in its own right. As time progressed it became increasingly clear that one individual or family could not hope to acquire all the skills needed to contribute to a civilised life – labour needed to be divided into groups. This process was greatly accelerated by the industrial revolution.

Today, we live in an age of increasing specialisation, and few nurses have the time or skills to mill their own flour or make their own cars! Increasingly, specialisation means that as new skills are acquired, old ones are either abandoned or relinquished to other specialists. We have all lost skills our grandparents took for granted, just as we have learned others which would have amazed them. Something is lost as something is gained, but on the whole, we, as individuals and as society are richer.

Nursing of course, is part of society, and the process of specialisation, of the loss and acquisition of skills, is mirrored within the profession. The increase in knowledge in our time has made, and will increasingly make it impossible for one nurse to acquire the information and skills required to practise generically – we are all specialists now. This presents us with both problems and opportunities. The central difficulty, it seems to me, is how increasingly specialised professions can respond to the need to treat the patient as a whole human being, how we can create effective helping strategies which recognise the patient as a thinking, feeling person who is an integral part of a complex network of relationships and a functioning member of society. I feel our best hope of resolving this dilemma in organisational terms lies in the mutidisciplinary team. This chapter will analyse the strengths and weaknesses of this approach, and reflect on ways to maximise the potential creativity of multidisciplinary working.

Communication and learning
Multidisciplinary team functioning depends on decisions being taken by the team as a whole, not exclusively by one or two powerful members. It requires open communication between all involved professionals, rather than the transmission of information and directives in one direction only.

The team approach requires the capacity to examine relationships between members in an honest, straightforward manner, and necessitates 'role blurring' – the capacity to relinquish rigid conceptions of one's own professional role, and a willingness to learn from others.

A policy or business meeting at which decisions affecting the team are made is a practical necessity and, to function effectively, this meeting must be genuinely democratic, allowing every member, however junior, to contribute to the decision making process. A clinical meeting at which workers are encouraged to share their work with others in a constructive environment is also desirable.

Patients should be allocated to staff on the basis of a careful assessment of the patient's needs, and a well thought out decision about which staff members have the specific skills required to meet those needs most effectively. In a community mental health team, for example, it would be appropriate for a patient with a clearly defined phobia to be referred to a worker with some training in behaviour therapy. However, a team member with no behavioural training might want to work as cotherapist, to acquire the necessary skills to work independently in future, or to prepare for further specialised training: this kind of cross fertilisation is one of the many benefits of multidisciplinary working.

Team meetings should be used to highlight the value of everyone's contribution – although the patient may need the services of different team members at different times, this does not imply that some are more valuable than others. Willingness to learn new skills from others and to pass on our own skills enhances rather than diminishes our professional integrity: it makes us better nurses.

Team members need to spend time getting to know each other if the team is to work effectively. Some teams find a sensitivity group, at which relationships between members can be frankly discussed, to be an effective way of resolving interpersonal problems. A group facilitator from outside the team should be sought if such a group is set up, and it should be made possible for all members to attend. Many teams also find it useful to set aside time occasionally for common group activities, such as policy review or shared learning. All these activities help to promote the team's cohesion and help it move towards a clearer formulation of its aims.

Problems and strategies

Occasionally, one or more workers may be unconvinced about the advantages of multidisciplinary working, or even opposed to it. This can present particular problems if the worker concerned is in a position of authority, such as a consultant. In the last resort, powerful staff members can, of course, prevent a multidisciplinary team from getting off the ground. This reality must be faced, but there are ways of preventing it.

A lengthy process of discussion and planning is necessary before a multidisciplinary approach is initiated, and the views of everyone involved need to be heard. The proposed philosophy needs to be specific, especially insofar as it relates to improved patient care and staff functioning. Much opposition to multidisciplinary working is based on misinformation which can be dispelled. The multidisciplinary approach cannot be imposed, nor can it be carried through by enthusiasm alone. However, managers and consultants are often prepared to tolerate multidisciplinary working if they feel the team knows what it is doing and they are kept informed of what is happening at every stage.

Just as all human groups contain the potential for creativity and cooperation, they also contain the potential for sterility and conflict. This need not be seen in a negative light – without conflict there can be neither learning nor growth for individuals or groups. A potent source of conflict in the team is the wide variety of professional backgrounds that members have, and from which they bring their preconceptions, assumptions and stereotyped attitudes. Traditional rivalries between the different professional groups is another complicating factor. By using team meetings to acquire understanding of how other members work, and encouraging role flexibility within the team, the worst effects of these often unconscious preconceptions can be mitigated. It is even possible for nurses to learn that doctors are capable of sensitivity and humility and for doctors to learn that nurses can take decisions!

Another problem can be posed by the different degrees of autonomy and specialisation to be found within any team. For example, a doctor, psychologist or social worker might be seen as having greater control over the quantity and kind of work she or he does than a community nurse. Although there is a certain amount of truth in this, it need not cause friction or lead nurses to devalue their own skills. All individuals bring something unique to their work, and a primary function of the multidisciplinary team is to assert the value of each individual within it.

Conflict can sometimes arise between the philosophy and practice of the team and the expectations of the professional hierarchies or institutions to which members also owe allegiance. Professional managers can feel threatened by a team over which they may feel they have little control while team members can feel insecure without the support of a professional hierarchy. Our own dependency needs enter into this: although we may not enjoy being told what to do, it is sometimes a comfort not having to think for ourselves. Again this difficulty is often more apparent than real. If regular meetings are held between the team and the relevant professional heads, and between members of particular professional groups within the team and their own managers, fantasies can be dispelled, anxieties reduced, and differences ironed out. Managers can also learn the advantages of allowing their subordinates a degree of autonomy, and team members those of developing their own resources and working more independently. Traditional hierarchical structures provide an element of security, while teamwork requires the ability to tolerate a certain amount of uncertainty – without it, professional and personal creativity becomes impossible.

Honest communication

In my experience, honest communication, whether of a positive or a constructively critical nature, does not occur between nurses as often as it should. Where it does occur, as it should in the multidisciplinary team, it can be unsettling because of its unfamiliarity. Constructive criticism of our work can feel like an attack, and we are often reluctant to engage in it ourselves for fear of upsetting colleagues or causing them to retaliate by criticising us. This attitude is misguided since it denies us the feedback necessary for change to take place – if we are not developing our full potential and are unaware of the fact, we need to hear it from our colleagues. This can happen without too much anxiety being aroused in the team meeting, where everyone is exposed to the same process. The emphasis throughout should be on the positive contribution each member makes, and mutual respect and goodwill are required.

Individuals within a team can sometimes find it difficult to tolerate unfamiliar ways of working in others and, if unchecked this can lead to a tendency towards sterile homogeneity. No two people are alike, and an emphasis on group cohesion at all costs can stifle individual initiative. Teams tend to fall into this trap if they feel exposed to external pressure, and meetings should expose and resolve any conflict. The team must not avoid its problems by imposing uniformity on its members.

Practical benefits

The team approach produces benefits for a very practical nature. Team members have a more accurate perception of their own and each others' skills than workers in hierarchical structures. This makes them less likely to take on work for which they are unfitted, and allows for more effective use of individual and team resources. It is much easier for multidisciplinary teams to arrive at an accurate assessment of patient needs, given the wide range of experience on which the team can draw, and to ensure a better 'fit' between the specific skills of team members and the specific needs of patients. An overwhelming advantage of this approach is that it resolves the dilemma of how to reconcile increasing specialisation with the need to provide a holistic model of care. Although the difficulties are formidable, its advantages both in terms of the development of team members' professional skills and the improvement in patient care make it well worth the trouble.

18

When disaster strikes: staff support after major incidents

Ian Woodroffe

Hospital Chaplain, Mayday Hospital, Thornton Heath, Surrey

Dealing with a major incident like a fire or a train crash can be an emotional experience for hospital staff. Feelings can range from excitement and interest to concern and grief. Following the Purley train crash, staff support groups were set up at the Mayday Hospital in Thornton Heath, and in giving support, they also gained understanding of staff reaction in this type of situation.

Calm atmosphere

Many staff members commented on how calm they felt while dealing with the initial emergency – some found this amazing among so many terrible injuries and so much suffering. Nursing staff were surprised by the manifestations of shock in many casualties, and felt overwhelmed by how 'good' people were. Despite their injuries, casualties constantly expressed concern for the trouble caused and apologised for being a nuisance. They also became irrationally concerned with detail, apologising for their dirty coat or asking where their other shoe was. Staff found these reactions overwhelming and difficult to understand.

Some staff members who live alone found the crash more difficult to cope with than those who have support at home. They found their journey home stressful, both due to the large scale of suffering they had witnessed and to not wishing to be at home alone. "I had to drive through Purley to get home," said one, "I felt sick when I arrived at an empty house."

Both male and female staff were prone to bursting into tears on the night of the crash, and for three to four days after – particularly on days three and four. Crying was often triggered by trivial incidents unconnected with the crash, and staff found these outbursts embarrassing, particularly in front of colleagues who had not dealt with the initial emergency, as they felt these colleagues would not understand.

Bad dreams

While some staff slept well on the night of the crash due to exhaustion, others could not 'switch off' either that night or the three or four after. Some had vivid and disturbing dreams about what they had seen – many full of anxiety for particular casualties. "I woke up suddenly shaking because I dreamt he had died. Even when I got to work and found he was still alive I had the same dream three days later," said one. On-call managers reported dreaming of a telephone ringing to summon them to another red alert situation.

Emotional reactions also had physical manifestations for some – one woman spoke of "sweating for three days", while others could not eat properly in the week after the crash, or reported starting to shake unexpectedly. These symptoms were discernible from around day three or four after the crash, and continued well into the following week.

Support staff
Reactions from staff not directly involved in caring for crash casualties were interesting. Catering staff felt they had something to offer (which was true), but also felt somewhat detached from the emergency. "We made piles of sandwiches, thinking they would be useful, but not really knowing whether or not they were needed." Chaplaincy volunteers were frustrated at having little to do – they had been sent home because "a lot of people have come in off the street to help, so we don't really need you." The volunteers felt a certain amount of rejection, having been involved with the hospital for years in some cases, yet not being allowed to help in this emergency. Secretarial staff taking calls from anxious relatives found it difficult to deal with them when they got rude and abusive.

The staff taking advantage of the support service after the crash came from many disciplines in the hospital, although no doctors or consultants did so. All reported feeling excited at being involved in a major incident, but also that it was not quite right to be excited about such a tragedy. A week after the crash, feelings were of job satisfaction and 'a job well done'. It seemed important to staff that their managers recognised this, and all said they had been well appreciated.

While there was an outward air of calm in all departments dealing with crash casualties, some people reported feelings of inadequacy, uselessness and helplessness. Others said they felt very alone among all the activity, and it is interesting to note that these people were the ones with managerial responsibility. One thing many staff found hard to accept was the fact that casualties were admitted to hospital with only a number to identify them, although the reasons for this were appreciated.

The following week
In the week after the crash, some staff who had not worked during the initial emergency felt guilty, and were unable to talk about it because of their guilt at 'not having done anything'. Those who had been present, on the other hand were snappy and impatient with colleagues. They felt isolated, a feeling carried over by some to their family and personal relationships, which were also affected by reactions to the crash. Many wanted to talk about their experiences, and felt unable to do so with

colleagues who had not been involved or with family and friends.

One thing the crash brought home to staff was how little they often know about patients after they are discharged. They reported feelings of unfinished business, and wanting to know how patients had progressed, or even what their name was, having only known them as a number.

Some staff felt they were expected to return to normal too quickly after the crash. Managers resented being expected to carry out a major organisational change 'imposed from above', only a few days after, and said this was insensitive. It was acknowledged that people need time to adjust to normal working patterns after such a major incident.

Reactions to the media among nurses were strong. While they were aware that casualties had consented to speak to reporters, nurses felt people's privacy was being invaded, and some doubted whether casualties should be asked to speak to the media so soon after an accident.

Dealing with staff reactions

The range of emotions staff can experience in the week or so after dealing with something like the Purley crash mean managers may need to consider giving them time off, or decreasing their workloads for a few days. If this is not possible, managers and colleagues should be aware that these staff may not be able to work to their usual standard for a time. It is also vital to acknowledge and give thanks for everyone's efforts in dealing with major incidents. This should not just include direct care staff – support staff who may not have been directly involved in patient care will also have put in extra effort and have felt some effects of the incident.

Recommendations

- Hospitals need a ready prepared support system for use after a major incident – possibly included in the major incident procedure document.
- Staff support systems should be available for everyday situations.
- Management need to be flexible with staff after a major incident.
- Reactions of staff following a major incident should be recorded, so that enough information can be collated for research into the subject.

The support exercise has shown us that major incidents like the Purley crash have a radical effect on staff involved – whether they are present at the initial emergency or not. While some staff were sceptical about the need for support groups, many needed to share their feelings with others who had been through the same thing. Some even said such support should be available to staff all the time. Hospitals would do well to have a prearranged staff support system set up for use immediately after such an incident – if support is not forthcoming quickly it is not as effective.

19

The Denford meeting – airing staff concerns

Janice Sigsworth, RGN
Formerly Senior Staff Nurse, The Charing Cross Hospital, London, now Ward Sister at University College Hospital, London

There are many factors in health care which can cause stress – the business of caring for ill people in itself can be stressful without the other problems of staffing, pay and communication and 'problem patients' which can crop up. A medical ward in the Charing Cross Hospital, London attempted to alleviate some of the factors causing stress among ward staff by holding a monthly meeting in which problems could be aired and difficulties with patients discussed.

The ward specialises in the care of breathless patients, and is staffed by two job sharing ward sisters, between eight and 12 registered nurses and eight to 12 student nurses. It is run on a primary nursing system, in which registered nurses care for a group of four to seven patients from admission through to discharge, working with other members of the multidisciplinary team.

The Denford meeting

The monthly meeting is known as the Denford meeting, named after Doctor John Denford, by whom it is chaired. Dr Denford is Director of the Cassel Hospital and a psychotherapist in patient community therapy. The meeting is chaired using a method described by Balint (1964). Research seminars had been organised at the Tavistock Clinic to study psychological implications in general medicine.

These seminars attempted to create a free, give and take atmosphere in which everyone could bring up their problems in the hope of gaining insight into them from the experience of others. The material for discussion at the Tavistock clinic was invariably provided by recent experiences with patients. It was essential for the group leader to refrain from making his own comments and criticisms until everyone had had ample time and space to express their thoughts.

As group leader in our meetings, Doctor Denford's role is to make his contributions ones which open up possibilities for the ward staff to discover for themselves some 'right' way of dealing with patient problems, rather than prescribing the right way to them.

The meeting takes place once a month, usually early on a Monday evening, and is held in the ward sitting room, unless patients are watching television, in which case it is held in the sister's office or an empty seminar room. The date of the meeting is publicised several days beforehand. The topic for discussion is decided by the doctors and nurses on the ward and, as suggested by Balint, is based on problems which arise when caring for patients. This is also publicised before the meeting, which usually lasts for an hour, with light refreshments provided by a nominated ward member – not always a nurse!

The meeting opens with brief, informal greetings as described by Balint. There is no reading from prepared reports or manuscripts – group members are asked to report freely on their experiences with the patients. Use of clinical notes is not encouraged but may be used as an aide-memoire. The aim is for group members to include as full an account as possible of their emotional responses to the problem, or even their emotional involvement in the patients' problems.

Such a frank account of the emotional aspects of the nurse/doctor-patient relationship can be obtained only if the atmosphere of the discussion is relaxed enough to enable group members to speak freely. Menzies (1960) states "The core of the anxiety situation for the nurse lies in her relationship with the patient. The closer and more concentrated this relationship the more likely the nurse is to experience the impact of anxiety, therefore the Denford meeting provides an excellent opportunity and environment to discuss and express these feelings." While a solution to the problem is often not found, staff are generally more aware of their own feelings and more clear about the needs of the patient.

Why is the meeting necessary?

As early as 1970 Menzies' attention was repeatedly drawn to the high level of tension and anxiety among nurses. The work situation arouses strong and mixed feelings in the nurse: pity, compassion, love, guilt, hatred and resentment towards the patients who arouse these strong feelings. Menzies examined the techniques employed by the nursing profession to contain and modify anxiety and hypothesised that nurses' struggle against anxiety can lead them to develop socially structured defense mechanisms such as restricted contact with patients through task allocation.

Kelly (1986) concluded in her study that patients who exhibit deviant behaviour are regarded as unpopular, which this supports Stockwell's theory (1984) that when nonconforming behaviour persists, patients come to be regarded as unpopular. Kelly recommended regular ward meetings to discuss difficulties with patients, and the purpose of the Denford meeting is to explore these feelings. Prior to the meetings, the patient who is causing problems has often been formally referred to the psychiatrist because they have been depressed or because members of the nursing or medical staff are concerned about the aspect of their behaviour.

Case study

George, aged 56, had been admitted to the ward six months previously for weight control, and was readmitted for the same reason. Two days following his readmission he suffered a right cerebral vascular accident. Prior to admission George was socially isolated. He had two female friends who appeared very overpowering, and he appeared to dislike them. He presented a number of problems to the nursing staff.

- He was sexually suggestive to the point of rudeness.
- He would not take his medicines when asked.
- He continually demanded food, telling several different nurses at different times that someone had taken his tray before he had finished.
- Initially he was very ill requiring physical nursing care, and was reluctant to become independent when he was over the acute stage.

During the Denford meeting at which George was the subject of discussion, it became obvious that he angered some staff with the disruptions he caused. Some felt sorry for him and wanted to help, but found this difficult because closeness was restricted by his sexual suggestions. Other nurses said he frustrated them or that they gave him one chance to take his medicines or to get out of bed – if he could not be bothered then neither could they and they would just leave him.

It became apparent that George demanded and got extra attention by all this destructive behaviour. For example, when giving George his medications, which would normally take two or three minutes, he would first refuse to take them, then say he would take them, then drop them on the floor which would require readministration and thus the saga continued. Coupled with this mounting anger and frustration, George appeared to give female members of the team more problems. He would have moments in which he would talk about his past life as a seaman and the places he had visited. This made many nurses feel guilty about their difficulties with him, because he showed that he could be a caring, intelligent person. A plan was formulated to overcome the problems George presented.

1. A day plan was drawn up, negiotated with George. This provided a united front so that if George demanded attention at an inappropriate time we could refer to the plan.
2. The problem posed by George's expression of his sexuality would be approached by two methods to meet the needs of the nurses:
   a. to confront him, telling him how difficult it was to be with him because of his comments;
   b. Some nurses felt they could not do this so they said they would ignore him when he made the comments but go to him at other times.

At the end of the meeting everyone felt optimistic about the plans to help staff cope with George and relieved that it was understandable to dislike George. As the reasons for his behaviour had become clear, however, the negative feelings towards him had subsided.

The Denford meetings give both nurses and doctors the chance to appreciate the difficulties and tensions in each other's work. The discussions allow people to share the troubles that difficult patients can cause, and give staff the chance to present a united front once plans are formulated. They are a useful and enjoyable way of reducing stress and, alleviating problems within patients that cause them to behave in a difficult manner.

References
Balint, M. (1964) The Doctor, His Patient and the Illness. Pitman, London.
Kelly, S. (1986) Nurses' perception of the Unpopular Patient. (Unpublished).
Menzies, I.E.P. (1970) Social Systems as a Defence Against Anxiety. Tavistock, London.
Stockwell, F. (1984) The Unpopular Patient. RCN, London.

Personal Freedom

20

Ensuring dignity and self esteem for patients and clients

Christine Morgan, RNMS, RGN

The author was Ward Sister, Bennetts End Hospital for the Mentally Handicapped, Hemel Hempstead, at the time that this chapter was written.

When I started training as a general nurse after working as a Registered Mental Handicap Nurse, several things struck me about the differences and similarities between the two care settings. I saw how vulnerable people become once they change from day clothes into pyjamas, and the impact of this on their self esteem, and I was also struck by the lengths to which designers had gone in the planning of general hospitals to ensure patient privacy was preserved, in total contrast to my experiences in institutions for mentally handicapped people. I knew that the dignity of mentally handicapped people is threatened by the attitudes of both the public and many care staff, and realised that these also prevail in general care and can affect patients similarly. These threats should be minimised for all patients, and nurses can have a major role in this. It is an essential aspect of nursing which I feel is frequently neglected.

Christine Morgan.

The dignity and self esteem of patients and clients must be uppermost in the mind of every nurse who assesses and plans care for their individual needs. Dignity and self esteem are closely linked (Figure 1): people can only behave with dignity if they have a reasonably good opinion of themselves, and their self-esteem depends, in part, on their freedom from conditions and situations which reduce their dignity.

Dignity: the state or quality of being worthy of honour or respect; sense of self-importance.

Self esteem: a good opinion of oneself.

When individuals from any social class or group are dependent on others to meet their living needs, a number of things threaten their dignity and self esteem. They also become very vulnerable once they change out of their day wear and into pyjamas. I wonder how many nurses are aware of this? Illness and physical weakness also increase this vulnerability. The impact of dependence and vulnerability on a person's dignity and self esteem is clearly much more profound for a long stay client.

Mentally handicapped people
The factors which threaten a person's dignity and self esteem may be even greater in both number and effect if that person is mentally handicapped. The nature of their handicaps (which may be multiple, and may include physical handicaps) may make it difficult for them to articulate their feelings and responses to the situation they are in, and may mean that they also have a particularly high degree of dependency on their carers, and for an indefinitely long period.

The attitudes of their carers and of society may reinforce their dependency, and actually limit their real capacity for independence. Someone who is treated as a child may have little motivation to behave and view themselves in any other way, even though they may be capable of more adult thought and action. The design of the buildings in which many mentally handicapped people live may also threaten their dignity and self esteem — the contrast between the design and facilities of a general hospital and those of many institutions for mentally handicapped people is very striking.

How can dignity and self esteem be preserved? With the development of systematic planning of individual patient care, nurses have become more aware of the need to consider the patient as a whole person, not only having an illness or handicap but also thoughts, feelings and opinions. Having and demonstrating respect for an individual reinforces his or her self esteem, and nurses play an important role in maintaining this by assessing an individual's needs and also his capabilities. The nurse can easily find out what the patient can do for himself and encourage him to do as much as his condition will allow.

'Personal' procedures
In the past, prior to an abdominal operation, patients were *given* a pubic shave; now nurses have started to question whether the person is capable of performing this for themselves, and if so, why they shouldn't be allowed to do so. The nurse could simply check to make sure that it is done thoroughly. This reduces embarrassment and a sense of helplessness on the part of the patient and also perhaps, that of a young and inexperienced junior nurse. Ensuring dignity and self esteem requires that the patient or client must have some say and control over what happens to him while he is in hospital, because 'self' esteem and 'self' worth are only achievable while he is actively involved, actively participating in his

own care. Relatives or close friends could also be involved more in the care of patients, perhaps with washing and dressing.

Privacy

Being forced to undergo certain procedures, or to eliminate or vomit without privacy is an intensely degrading situation for most people. Provision for privacy is generally much better in most general hospitals than in most institutions for mentally handicapped people. In many general hospitals designers and planners have gone to great lengths to ensure that patients' privacy is preserved. Wards are cubicalised; there are usually sufficient bathrooms and showers, even bidets in some wards; also numerous toilets; some patients have single rooms, and there are screens around beds to give added privacy. There may be treatment rooms on all wards, where patients can have dressings changed and removed privately.

In most hospitals for mentally handicapped people, facilities are much poorer. Toilets are not cubicalised and often have no doors; bathroom doors don't have locks; some have no doors at all; there may be a large number of clients having to share the one bathroom and there is often no place for clients to dress and undress in private. These problems are very much structural and not readily changed by the nurse. But this lack of provision for privacy should not lead anyone to assume that it is therefore not important to their clients, and more strenuous efforts are required to ensure some privacy despite the lack of available resources.

Elimination Many patients become constipated, partly as a result of their inactivity but also due to their acute embarrassment at having to perform a very private activity in a 'public' place. The nurse should consider allowing the patient to go to the toilet once he is mobile enough, possibly helping him there and back, and should also put a mobile screen in front of the toilet or bathroom entrance to give it the sense of privacy, if it lacks a door.

Effective communication If the details of procedures are explained to the patient beforehand, he will be much better prepared for what is to come, and the fact that the nurse respects his need for this information supports his self esteem. It is important, for example, before passing a nasogastric tube, to explain what one is going to do, why, and what the patient will experience, and also to discuss how he can help in the procedure.

Feeding Many mentally handicapped clients have multiple handicaps — some are physically disabled and blind. What can be worse than being fed without knowing from which direction the spoon is coming; what is on the spoon, and being unable to say they don't like what is being given? It is essential to communicate with the client, tell him what is being given, encourage him to hold the spoon, so he is aware of it and knows it is not just going to arrive at his mouth apparently from nowhere.

This communication demonstrates the nurse's respect for the patient, contributes to raising his opinion of himself and also gives him some control over what happens to him.

Living space and style of dress Recent research (Blunden, 1985) has shown that simply allowing patients to display their own belongings, giving them their own living space, and involving them in decision-making on changes in their environment, brings about a marked improvement in their apparent dignity and consequently their attitude towards care.

In mental handicap hospitals, simple and inexpensive measures can be taken, such as arranging existing furniture in such a way as to allow the client some control over an area he can recognise as his own living space. Encouraging him to have his own belongings, to display pictures, and if possible to have his own front door key; arranging the decor of living areas and also his style of dress in ways appropriate to his age will all contribute to the individual's dignity and self esteem.

Ensuring dignity and self esteem

Many features of illness, handicap and of the various settings for care and essential clinical procedures potentially threaten an individual's dignity and self esteem.

Much of the freedom, and many of the everyday experiences which we take for granted, have to be compromised and modified if we are ill, or become handicapped in some way. The dependence we must then place on others deprives us of some of the control we normally expect to have over our own lives.

Perhaps the most important question we as nurses should ask ourselves about our patients and clients is: 'would I accept this situation for myself, a friend or relative?' If the answer is 'no' then we must take steps to improve the care we give, and the environment in which our patients and clients live. Most of all, we need, at all times, to respect them as individual people.

NB Throughout this chapter the male gender has been used to refer to all patients and clients, but is intended to include both male and female patients and clients.

Bibliography
Blows, H. and Alcoe, J. (1985) Lifestyles for people with mental handicap. E.S.C.A.T.A.
    A staff training exercise based on the principle of normalisation.
Blunden, R. (1980) Individual plans for mentally handicapped people. Mental Handicap Applied Research Unit, Wales.
    A guide to implementing individual programme plans for mentally handicapped people.

Chilman and Thomas (1981) Understanding Nursing Care, Second Edition. Churchill Livingstone, Edinburgh.
    A textbook designed to help learners and qualified nurses to develop a sympathetic and perceptive approach to care.
Elliott, J. and Bayes. K. (1972) Room for Improvement: a better environment for the mentally handicapped. King Edward's Hospital Fund for London.
    This discusses the ways in which simple, cost effective measures and attention to design can create a more homely and therapeutic environment for mentally handicapped people in both in and out of hospital.
English National Board, (1985) Caring for people with Mental Handicap. ENB, London.
    This package for learners is based on the 1982 syllabus for the RNMS course.

References
Blunden, R. (1985) A New Style of Life: a study of the impact of moving into an ordinary house on the lives of mentally handicapped people. Mental Handicap Applied Research Unit, Wales.
Hanks, P. (Editor) (1979). Collins Dictionary of the English Language. William Collins Sons and Co Ltd, Glasgow.

21
Respecting clients' dignity

Jo Yeats, RNMH
Staff Nurse, Tatchbury Mount, Calmore, Nr Totton, Hants.

Historically, large institutions were built to provide custodial care for mentally handicapped people which, until recently, was seen as the only possible approach. Individual dignity, self-esteem or independence of the patients were not issues worthy of consideration.

Long, overcrowded dormitories, locked doors, lack of personal privacy and various forms of punishment were regarded as quite normal and segregation of mentally handicapped people from the rest of the community was a matter of course.

These societal beliefs and attitudes led to the denial not only of the services and freedom enjoyed by the rest of the community but to the denial of all basic human rights.

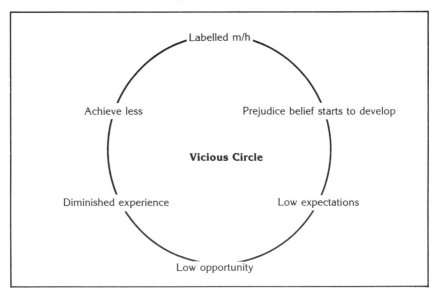

Figure 1. Devaluation Model.

Inherited attitudes

Prejudice still exists against many types of people, not only those with a mental handicap. Labels such as 'punk', or 'the unemployed', lead to whole groups becoming devalued as members of society. Common and often untrue beliefs, founded on fear and ignorance, have been passed down through the generations.

In the past, autocratic decisions were taken about groups of people seen as problems to society, rather than any attempt being made to meet individual need. People with a mental handicap were regarded as unsafe or possessed by the devil, best dealt with in segregation.

Towards the end of the last century, a popular public diversion was to visit the local asylum to view the 'lunatics', where the behaviour of the wretched, untreated inmates confirmed such beliefs.

Such low opinions, which still lurk in many areas of the public consciousness, lead to low expectations of mentally handicapped people. There is therefore little or no opportunity created for them to find a role in society, or for individuals to realise potential ability (Figure 1).

The Jay Report

In 1979, the Jay Committee, chaired by Peggy Jay, put forward proposals to improve the quality of life for those afflicted with a mental handicap and to begin the lengthy process of changing public attitudes. It stated: "Mentally handicapped people have the right to be treated as individuals, to live life to the full and to have access to the same services as 'normal people'."

It went on to say that staff employed should have the "right qualities and attitudes."

These recommendations should be regarded as a blueprint for future planning to promote better living conditions and environments. Some changes have already taken place. Huge institutions are giving way to small family houses and hospital wards are being humanised by allowing the residents to exercise free choice of colours and furnishings. These changes have affected not only the people with a mental handicap but those who care for them, thus preserving the dignity and self-esteem of both groups. The United Nations Declaration of Rights for Disabled Persons (Williams and Shoultz, 1982) states: "Disabled persons have the inherent right to respect for their human dignity." As an employee I believe we must have total respect for the individuals with whom we work to ensure their needs are fully met.

Normalisation

As a philosophy of care, 'normalisation' must come to the fore if carers are to believe and put into practice the principle that people with a mental handicap should have equal opportunity to experience activities enjoyed by their peers. It means improved freedom of choice, and wider participation in many activities with a view to enriching their lifestyle.

Hierarchy of human needs

Each individual must be appreciated as a unique person with a set of specific needs. In 1970, Maslow (Clarke, 1982) identified the Hierarchy of Human Needs (Figure 2). This demonstrates that everyone has basic physical needs which must be fulfilled before the person can seek to meet the next areas of need in ascending order.

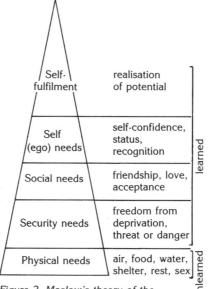

Figure 2. Maslow's theory of the hierarchy of needs.

For each person there are other specific needs and absolute levels of achievement within each layer of this structure. To help a person reach his or her highest possible potential they must be given opportunities to practise until that level of competence is acquired.

For someone with a mental handicap, this could mean gaining complex skills for employment or more basic daily living skills. Respect for a person's beliefs and rights as a human being help to build confidence and generate a high degree of motivation.

Until recently, people with a mental handicap were denied freedom of speech, and therefore self advocacy was impossible. It has been defined as: "... speaking or acting for yourself. It means deciding what is best for you and taking charge of getting it. It means standing up for your rights as a person." (Williams and Shoultz, 1982). Skills that need to be taught include knowledge of individual rights, how to value yourself, make decisions and fight for what you believe is right. Many of these skills can be taught — the issues don't have to be large. For example, someone who has lived in a large institution can learn he has the right to a quiet drink at the local pub.

Society's attitudes can only be changed slowly by education. Gradual integration rather than segregation of people with a mental handicap is called for. They must have the same right to education, employment and housing as non-handicapped people enjoy. If society can recognise that they are 'people first', then the concept of integration into the community, respecting the dignity of each individual, would become a reality.

Bibliography
Atkinson, R.L., Atkinson, R.C. and Hilgard, E.R. (1983) Introduction to Psychology. Harcourt Brace, Jovanovich International Edition.
Bogdand, R. and Taylor, S.J. (1982) Inside Out. University of Toronto Press. Clarke, D. (1982) Mentally Handicapped People. Balliere Tindall, London.
Jay, P. et al (1979) Report of the Committee of Enquiry into Mental Handicap Nursing and Care. HMSO, London.
McConkey, R. and McCormack (1983) Breaking Barriers. Souvenir Press (E and A Ltd).
Williams, P. and Shoultz, B. (1982) We can speak for ourselves. Souvenir Press (E and A Ltd).
Williams, P. and Shoultz, B. (1982) Technical Assistance for Self Advocacy Work Book.

22

Labelling: attitudes, beliefs and customs

Gillian James, RNMH, RGN, RCNT, FE Teacher Cert
Nurse Teacher, Department of Continuing Education, Brent House, Hatton, Warwickshire and also Vice Chairman, RCN Society of Mental Handicap Nurses

In 1986 at the Annual Meeting of the Royal College of Nursing Representative Body, a resolution was passed by a large majority asking RCN Council to take appropriate action to raise the level of public awareness about the special needs of people with mental or physical handicap. The labelling theory was used in support of the argument and it was emphasised that real effort should be made to avoid over-professionalism and to develop a more appropriate image for this group of people who are, after all, our fellow citizens and entitled to be treated as such.

Following the debate, I felt there was a need to increase not only *public* awareness but awareness within the nursing profession about the whole concept of labelling, how it is used and what effects it has.

Attitudes to labelling

In her book, Shearer (1981) says it is the inability of people which leads to labelling. Everyone has setbacks, she asserts, but disablement means having to face problems every day. She questions what makes them the disabled population. Is it where they live? Where they go to school? Where they spend their adult life? Do others set up special requirements and laws for them? If so, does this make their disability more conspicuous? Does it mean that they cannot cope with the term 'normal life'? Are we tolerant enough of human weaknesses? As the health of the general population improves, do we view any deformity, however small, with contempt or intolerance?

Spencer (1977) looks at terminology and says terms "reflect the hopes and fears, the precepts, prejudices, ignorance, arrogance, optimism and pessimism".

Myers and Heron (1985) state: "It is the way in which and the extent to which the needs of the intellectually impaired and thereby disabled person are or are not met that determines the degree to which he or she is handicapped." They go on to say that the perception of people with intellectual disability as being capable of learning may not be held by those in society who have a major say in providing resources. The disabled person may develop a poor self-image and show incompetence in several areas of development. The problem is mostly one of attitudes.

A person with a mental handicap who, for instance, has shown severe behaviour disorder, has often been segregated or even moved to a more secure place. If they have committed an offence they will be relabelled, for example, under a section of the 1983 Mental Health Act as being mentally handicapped, having a behaviour problem and needing control under the law. The restriction placed on them may accord even more prejudiced attitudes upon that person.

Does this mean that the consequences of labelling and blame for the existence of subculture lies with those who have the power to control and are agents of change within the social framework of the nation? What are the consequences of labelling, how does it happen and how can it be avoided?

The labelling theory

According to theorists who have studied labelling, it is the labelling of a person which ensures his behaviour. The label not only does this but also reinforces his behaviour until it becomes an identifiable and perhaps permanent feature of that person. In the medical sense it is the punitive labelling to which society reacts and defines the unacceptable behaviour as 'deviant'. The label defines that person as being of a particular kind and the tendency is to interpret what he does in terms of the label.

Labelling is also class-linked. Members of lower status groups appear to have a lower resistance to particular stigmatising labels. Attitudes to the same behaviour in two different social groups will be treated in two different ways. For example, a group of youngsters seen fighting in lower income groups would be interpreted as being of low intellectual level. The same situation in a wealthy area would be treated as high spiritedness. Race is also often used in a similar way as a social labelling device (Rack, 1982).

Stigma

Some groups have the power to make labels stick, namely the professional groups; the police, the courts, teachers, social workers and nurses, for example. The labelling of a person or a group does not remain neutral; it overrides any other status that person has. Others may respond to him in terms of that particular label and not to him as an individual. Stigma probably also reinforces what would otherwise have been a short-lived behaviour, people tend to have expectations of that person's behaviour and so label him.

The label will then encapsulate the total condition in the eyes of others and identify that person or group, often to the detriment of other areas in their total make-up. The person is then classed as a 'deviant' and is socially sanctioned or treated as such with the label concerned with the negative definition of him.

Any behaviour which is not socially accepted is then selected for special attention and even highlighted because a person has a stigmatising label. The same behaviour may well go unnoticed or overlooked in the rest of society, but the labelled person may be punished or penalised (Haralambos, 1985). The label may often deny that person the right to live an ordinary life, a right which is open to most people.

Because of this, a subculture develops and within this the attitudes, values and beliefs identifying the group justify its existence and support its activities. In fact, those within that subculture often act within the terms of the concept of the group, and society itself applies pressure to the group or individual to be treated as they are labelled. The label may well be retained well into adulthood and the individual qualities of that person overlooked because of the clinical diagnosis of his condition which defines how he will function.

Irreversible

Owens and Birchenall (1979) described labelling as a "global one and once a person becomes labelled it is often almost always irreversible. Labelling affects a person's self-esteem. Some may even adopt a 'cover' story in order to cope with it.

"A labelled person can be defined in some way as standing in opposition to the normal society (placed outside and made to feel 'strange').

"Stigmatisation is an important aspect of labelling as people will often react to differences in speech, sight, hearing or physical features; this will become uppermost in their mind and they will react by either being able to interact with them or retreating.

"This reaction will often be dependent on that person's exposure to the disability and by how much experience they have had in the past. Labelling has sometimes been thought of in the past as being in the best interests of the disabled person, often when it has then been required to have treatment, special care or training."

Trying to solve the issue of labelling

If labelling comes about because our beliefs and attitudes colour the way we see situations that present problems, we must carefully judge our attitudes as professionals. Do patients admitted to hospital adopt the role required of them because of the function of that place? Are institutions both within and outside the NHS equal to regulations, bureaucracy, conformity, uniformity (Hockey, 1981)?

Does society highlight the disabilities by having special declarations of rights, Ministers for the Disabled, Mental Health Acts and special categories within the welfare system?

In its leaflet, the Campaign for People with a Mental Handicap (CMH)

(1987) lists commonplace misconceptions of mental handicap:

- Mental handicap is hereditary.
- Mental handicap is the same as being mentally ill.
- People with a mental handicap cannot speak for themselves.
- They cannot look after themselves.
- They can be violent, dangerous and unpredictable.
- There will always be some who need to live in hospital
- They prefer to be with their own kind.
- People do not want those with a mental handicap in their street... anyway it lowers the property values...

Community care

When developing community care and looking at, for example, strategies for coping with different types of handicapping conditions, any changes need to be done with a great deal of sensitivity. The public reaction to handicapping conditions may well reduce the chances of that service succeeding. Prejudices and therefore rejection are often a result of a lack of knowledge and understanding.

Terminology often does not help and the use of words such as 'mental patient' often describes quite wrongly and inappropriately those who have been in hospitals or institutions perhaps for many years, when in fact they do not require hospital treatment.

When providing community care for those who have lived in institutional settings with their rules and regulations, a great deal of re-education has to take place both for the resident and the general public. Being labelled an ex-patient often makes re-entry into the community quite difficult. Do disabled people, and in particular people with a mental handicap, fit into the community as a member of that society? Are they accepted or does the stigma of having once lived in an institution follow them into the new setting?

One way of solving the problem and stopping the stereotyping may well be to accept the label but change the negative association of it to a positive one, and not allow it to colour other statuses that person may have. If the label is accepted then perhaps some of the presenting features of the condition may also be accepted.

Nursing staff can play an important role in all aspects of disablement and handicaps. It is essential that reactions of members of a family into which a handicapped child is born are very carefully responded to by the professionals, particularly the nurses who are involved in the delivery and early part of that child's life.

The responses by the parents must be fully understood in order that they are coped with expertly; nurses play an important part in supporting that family through each crisis. If the physical features of a person are part of the label, they may identify a specific condition, syndrome or diagnosis but this may also suggest, for example, a life expectancy which causes a great deal of anxiety for the parents.

We need to look at the disabled person not as someone with a physical or mental affliction but as a whole person with individual needs, and to build up their self-esteem. A change in terminology could help but "if real advances are to be made, community programmes need to include a more 'normal' living environment" (Owens and Birchenall, 1979). Everyone should be a valued member of society. This can only be achieved if people with a mental handicap are seen as part of the local community. For this to happen, adequate services and resources are essential to give them the opportunities other people take for granted.

Bibliography

Craft, M. et al (1985) Mental handicap – A Multidisciplinary Approach. Bailliere Tindall, Eastbourne.
An excellent textbook on mental handicap.
Heron, A. and Myers, M. (1983) Intellectual Impairment – the Battle Against Handicap. Academic Press, London.
These co-authors are well known within all disciplines in mental handicap.
Parrish, A. (1987) Essentials of Nursing – Mental handicap. Macmillan Education, Basingstoke.
A new book in the series.
Parsons, T. (1951) The Social System. Free Press of Glencoe, New York.
The author is a well known, often quoted sociologist.
Scheff, T. (1966) Being Mentally Ill – a Sociological Theory. Aldine Press, Chicago.
This broadens the discussion to include mental illness.
Sugden, J. (1985) Labelling theory. *Nursing,* **2,** 35, 1021.
A good article, specifically on labelling.
University of Kent (1987) (PSSRU) People First. Care in Community Newletter, 7, 11.
The Personal Social Services Research Unit is currently studying mental handicap relocation projects.
Warnock Committee Report (1978) Special educational needs. Cmnd 7212, HMSO, London.
This report recommends 'special' education for children regarding labelling.

References

CMH (1987) Campaigning for valued futures with people who have learning difficulties: Fact and fallacies. CMH, London.
Haralambos, M. (1985) Sociology – Themes and Perspectives. University Tutorial Press, Slough.
Hockey, L. (1981) Current Issues in Nursing. Churchill Livingstone, Edinburgh.
Mental Health Act (1983) HMSO, DHSS.
Myers, M. and Heron, A. (1985) Concepts about Mental Handicap. *Physiotherapy,* **71,** 3, 102-4.
Owens, G. and Birchenall, P. (1979) Mental Handicap – the Social Dimensions. Pitman Medical Publications, Tunbridge Wells.
Rack, P. (1982) Race, Culture and Mental Disorder. Tavistock Press, London.
Shearer, A. (1981) Disability – Whose Handicap? Blackwell, Oxford.
Spencer, D.A. (1977) What's in a name? *Apex,* **5,** 1, 102.

23

Are we handicapped by our sexual prejudices?

Amanda Gunner, RNMH, DipN, CertEd, RNT
Senior Tutor, Waltham Forest School of Nursing, London

Sexuality is a human function which causes a great deal of embarrassment. The strength of feeling and the need to impose our own personal relationships are one part of sexuality most of us have experienced. However, society seeks to deny its relevance to a man or woman with a mental handicap. This article seeks to explore how as carers, whether parents or professionals, we have made valued judgements upon men and women who have a mental handicap, especially with regard to their personal relationships. It is not an account of how to teach or facilitate a sex education programme. Long before such a project could be undertaken, we, the carers must be clear about the notions of choice and personal freedom, especially as part of living in the latter end of the twentieth century means that relationships are viewed as symbols of success. We are continually bombarded by the media with 'answers' to help us strive for the ideal. Advertising with its suggestive overtones pressurises us into believing success is synonymous with being cared for and loved. If however, you are unable to participate in the relationships game, then to a greater or lesser extent you may be rejected by society. This pressure has not, however, been matched by a change in the strong taboos associated with discussing sexual relationships and other intimacy. We need to be clear, and to free ourselves from the use of euphemisms if we are to communicate effectively and sensitively on the subject. As advocates and carers, we need to resolve the issue within ourselves before we can work effectively and progress in this important part of human life.

Role of the carer

The fundamental premise is that society (not just Ms Average, but carers and professionals) cannot cope with the idea that disabled people have the same needs and desires as themselves. The whole area of socio-sexual education can become an unmanageable task.

People with a mental handicap have difficulties in learning. Our role is to teach and facilitate learning to take place. Kempton (1980) distinguishes between **understanding** and **behaviour.** The following example highlights this difference.

"Many people do not understand in any detail how their car engine works; but that lack of understanding does not stop them driving thousands of miles each year, and acting appropriately by observing the rules of the road, periodically checking oil, tyre pressure and petrol, filling up where necessary. The **understanding** component is very small compared to the behaviour or **do** component" (Craft, 1987).

All kinds of relationships are based on communication. This need to communicate with other human beings in one way or another can be restricted for a person with mental handicap. They have not been given the right to know, either because of the protective environment in which they live or due to their own particular circumstances.

Devising a suitable programme of sex education for people with a mental handicap is not simply a case of looking at what the client requires, although this is of paramount importance. Socio-sexual education is about attitudes of both teacher and student – how, as a teacher, we enable the man or woman with a mental handicap to explore and understand their feelings, themselves and the behaviour they use to help and sometimes protect them.

People's attitudes

Attitudes of the carers, whether parents or professionals, tend to exhibit behaviour that says either 'I don't want to be involved' or 'I will control'. Non-involvement is the Victorian attitude we do not talk about this, it is shameful and therefore should be kept secret. The control aspect is no better. Superficially there may be some discussion about sexuality but it is about conformity, not choice. Both reactions are extreme, and to find a middle line that is not mediocrity requires care and sensitivity.

As carers we must identify the factors involved when looking at sexual relationships. There are at least four factors involved:

- Your own attitude towards sex.

- The perception of your own child as a sexual being.

- Your own concept of sex education.

- Your own use of language when discussing sexual matters.

We all have sexual feelings which may be satisfied, denied, suppressed, impulsive or destructive. This list immediately highlights a number of negative views about sex which may then distort our attitude towards it.

Again, throughout the media we hear about and see constantly unwanted pregnancies; family violence; incest; rape and sexual assault. It is easy to believe that sexual feelings are urges which should be restrained and that for people with a mental handicap they should be stopped. This view is still commonplace even when from both the literature available and our own experiences, "we know that sexual development in persons our society designates as mildy and moderately retarded, broadly follows the normal pattern" (Heshusius, 1987).

A parent's view

The experience of parents perceiving their child as a sexual being is summed up accurately by a parent of a daughter with a mental handicap. Pauline Fairbrother (1983) asks: "why do parents in particular, become so depressed and worried at the first signs of sexual awareness, whether it is masturbation or giggling at someone of the opposite sex or becoming curious about their body? We should welcome joyously these signs as yet another manifestation of the normality of our son or daughter. The things that they have in common with the rest of us are far more numerous than the things that are different."

The professional's view

Nurses and other care staff are often no better than those worried parents. One of a number of studies carried out to look at acknowledgement by care staff of the sexual needs of people with a mental handicap stated that "of staff questioned, one quarter of nurses in institutions, and one fifth of hostel staff thought that adult residents should be discouraged from developing sexual relationships" (Jay, 1978). This appears to be the most recent study in Britain, and hopefully the attitudes reported are a little dated. However, it seems, in the light of a case in 1987 in which the House of Lords agreed with both the Court of Appeal and a High Court Judge, in sanctioning the sterilisation of a 17 year-old girl with a mental handicap, nearly a decade since the Jay report, that there is still little progress in maintaining human rights for people with a mental handicap. We seem to be no nearer an enlightened society.

Sexual needs

The notion of sex education is, wrongly, of tangible, clinical procedure, nothing to do with developing relationships and the bonding that takes place sexually between two people. The warmth and enjoyment is excluded, the reason for sex education is seen as the elimination of sexual abuse and disease. People with a mental handicap are vulnerable and need more than a sex education programme. So often the most personal needs of a man or woman with a mental handicap must be dealt with by another person. This, coupled with the need to conform with the routines of the institution or family, leave the person with little or no control over their own body and with poor self-esteem.

Coping with possible sex abuse is about knowing your rights, having had the chance to experience relationships and know how to react and behave. Ignorance is not bliss, it is dangerous.

"A great deal of unhappiness and ill health can result for those who fail to manage their relationships successfully. Marital partners, friends, kin and workmates are all extremely important in different ways" (Argyle and Henderson, 1985). Becoming sexually aware needs support and intimacy of varying degrees, but not one of us could complete the course of life without the help of others. Sexuality is a human function, and one which we all have the right to express.

Remember the **understanding** component of how a car works? Few of us have that, or the ability to understand sexual needs. Most of us have our vision clouded by the ideal, a romantic idea that hinders developing our own, or anyone else's, social skills in forming relationships. No-one expects any of us to be continually successful when getting to know people. Why then should we expect men and women with a mental handicap to have to strive for perfection? This, coupled with a lack of risk taken by people with control over their lives makes their relationships limited. There are no opportunities for many to choose how far a particular relationship will proceed or the way in which it will happen.

Not only do we lack understanding of sexuality, but also that of personal freedom. The right of people with a mental handicap to have relationships is being addressed to some degree, but their right to choose from the full gambit of varying levels of sexuality and relationships is being conveniently pushed to one side.

As carers, parents, or professionals we advocate the rights of people with a mental handicap. This is not enough. We need to understand the notion of personal freedom. The choice to take risks within relationships is an important need within us all. When will we begin to show men and women with a mental handicap that freedom and choice is for them to explore and not for us to confine?

References

Argyle, M. and Henderson, M. (1985) The Anatomy of Relationships; and the rules and skills needed to manage them successfully. Heinemann, London.

Craft, A. (1987) Mental Handicap and Sexuality. Costello, London.

Heshusius, L. (1987) Research and perceptions of sexuality by persons labelled mentally retarded. In: Craft, A. (1987) previously cited.

Kempton, W. (1980) Sex Education for Persons with Disabilities that hinder learning (2nd Ed) Philadelphia Planned Parenthood Association of South Eastern Pennsylvania. In: Craft A. (1987) previously cited.

Jay, P. (1978) Report of the Committee of Enquiry into Mental Handicap Nursing and Care. (CMND 7468-11). HMSO, London.

24

Informed consent: a patient's right?

Alison Kennett, RGN, Cert. Onc
Research Sister, Royal Marsden Hospital, Surrey

Nurses involved in patient education all face the decision of what information should and should not be disclosed. The boundaries of patient advocacy are unclear and nursing ethics must play a part in providing guidelines for what is divulged. In areas such as oncology nursing, the issue of informed consent is particularly important and should be discussed.

Research has shown that the more knowledge patients have about their disease and its subsequent treatment, the more they are able to participate in their own care and the better they feel, both mentally and physically (Hayward, 1973). This research is related specifically to postoperative patients but from my experience in oncology this statement is still most relevant. Indeed it is used on the inside cover of the Royal Marsden Hospital patient education booklet series on all subjects relating to cancer. But the problems arise when we consider who should tell patients, what they should be told, when it should be told and also where it should be told.

Before a patient receives any care it is essential to obtain an informed consent. Failure to do so can give rise to both civil and criminal proceedings (Martin, 1977).

What is informed consent?

A doctrine of informed consent has evolved and patients' rights, as established in the doctrine, have direct implications for the nursing profession collectively and individually. By law, no diagnostic or therapeutic procedure can be performed on a patient without him having been told the risks of the procedure and the alternatives to it prior to giving his consent (Bucklin, 1975). As far back as 1914 Judge Cardozo declared that "every human being of adult years and sound mind has a right to determine what should be done with his or her own body". The principle of informed consent is derived from Anglo-American law which holds that an individual is master over his own body and, if mentally competent, may choose to refuse even life-saving treatment. The United States has much published material on the whole issue of informed consent, whereas English sources are much less abundant. No doubt this is due to the fact that America has substantial legislation in this area, particularly the Patients' Bill of Rights which includes many of the elements listed below.

Elements of informed consent The essential elements of informed consent should include:

- a full explanation of the proposed treatment involving important incidental procedures;
- information in a manner intelligible to the patient involving as little jargon as possible;
- explanation of inherent risks and benefits;
- alternatives to proposed treatment;
- adequate time to allow the patient to question the proposals, to ensure the patient realises he has the option to withdraw consent from the treatment or procedure whenever he likes — indeed he has the right to refuse any treatment initially.

Obtaining informed consent

There appear three difficult areas in obtaining a meaningful consent:
　i)who should give the information?
　ii)what information should be disclosed?
　iii)where should the information be given?

Both Miller (1980) and Bucklin (1975) state that it is the doctor's responsibility to provide enough information to his patients so that an intelligent decision about the procedure can be made. Barkes (1978) also says that disclosure for consent should be regarded as the doctor's prerogative as he is the one to perform the procedure and his is the ultimate responsibility for the communication of facts. In most cases it is the doctor who obtains the consent but in some incidences it may be the senior nurse who obtains the signature on the form after the doctor has explained the procedure.

Besch (1979) in investigating the possible barriers to obtaining a meaningful consent, found that the doctor-patient relationship appeared to interfere with patient autonomy. The patient tended to trust the doctor's recommendation completely and many did not understand that it was a choice that was being asked of them and not complete compliance. Comments such as these illustrate this: ''I guess the doctor knows best.'' ''I wasn't going to argue with him, he knows what he is doing.'' ''If that's what you think I should do, doctor.''

Surely, by virtue of this authoritative role, the physician may, inadvertently, introduce an element of coercion into the consent procedure, thus preventing the patient from making a voluntary decision. ''Coercion nullifies consent'' (Meissel, 1977).

Effective communication

''Doctors often find it difficult to relax with patients who have incurable cancer and this impairs their ability to communicate effectively with them''

(Hanks, 1983). It must be here that the creation of a patient advocate position would be enormously beneficial to ensure the patient's comprehension of the medical information before making a decision. The nurse can amplify, clarify and encourage questioning if the doctor has used jargon-laden phrases and shrouded the true message sufficiently to render a patient unclear as to what the doctor is actually explaining. I feel that it is the nurse who may be more skilled and more aware of non-verbal cues and other communication techniques. She is constantly at hand to answer any subsequent questions that may be posed by the patient, whereas the doctor is likely to be off the ward most of the time and only contactable by going through the time consuming bleep system.

The nurse herself has to be well informed and perceptive in order to assess the extent of the patient's comprehension. This will only come as a result of an established rapport with the patient with whom the nurse has had most contact and who, I suggest, has the patient's wishes foremost in her mind.

What to disclose
Wells (1979) stated that "In the treatment of malignant disease it is often at diagnosis that a catalogue of deceit and half-truths begins, when those whose responsibility it is fail to be honest with the patient and the members of the health care team become entangled with the complicated task of keeping information from the patient."

This makes a mockery of obtaining subsequent informed consent for necessary procedures. Another problem is that explanation is time consuming and some physicians would argue that full explanations produce unwarranted anxiety. It is known, however, that explicit information prior to a procedure can lead to a substantially improved prognosis. "Is it then ethical or fair to decide without the patient's knowledge what he should or should not know about his own life? Is it right to assess a personality, and its potential, without knowledge of its strengths and weaknesses, after a brief contact arranged for an entirely different purpose? The position is rather similar to knowing that an individual is going to have to perform a task requiring considerable fortitude and endurance. The individual is kept in ignorance of the true nature of the task on the grounds that it is best not to anticipate an unpleasant experience, so that the individual is shocked and unprepared for what then transpires" (Goldie, 1982).

Alternative treatments
Alternative treatments may not be proposed to the patient, who remains unaware of the options. Interestingly, a nurse who was practising in the United States of America, where there is a Patients' Bill of Rights ensuring that they have the right of self determination, chose to explain to a patient alternative methods of treatment available which a doctor had not, and was found guilty of professional misconduct — a decision against which

she is now appealing. Here an ethical argument arises; the nurse, acting as informer of the alternative treatment, presents an ethical dilemma involving her in the actual decision for the planned treatment whereas the doctor is more removed from the emotional aspect of the decision-making.

Where the information is given The circumstances in which information is presented are often overwhelming — the patient is usually in hospital, in unfamiliar surroundings with strangers around, being confronted with procedures to undergo and invasions of privacy. Often the information is given implying that the decision is required immediately and the patient does not appear to have an opportunity to discuss the proposals. Nurses are rarely present when surgeons or physicians explain the reasons for, and what is involved in surgical and medical procedures. This "right hand not knowing what the left hand is doing" syndrome confuses both nurses and patients and may have a disastrous impact on the patient's overall trust in the caring team. While it would be wrong to suggest many forms of consent are obtained without the patient being fully aware of his illness and its likely outcome, it would be equally wrong to pretend it does not happen.

"It is in situations such as these that a nurse is required to support her colleagues and assure the patient. Can the nurse be expected to support the decision that a patient is to have further surgery in the hope of curing what is known to all except the patient to be an incurable disease?" (Wells, 1982).

The values of effective communication between patient and carer seem easy to state but difficult to put into action. It involves a commitment to patients' rights to decide what happens to their own bodies. To uphold such views health professionals, especially doctors, must learn to become more communicative and less paternalistic and they must accept that informed consent is an essential part of the doctor-patient-nurse relationship and of proper patient care. The nurse's role as patient intermediary requires knowledge and a commitment to this concept of assisting patients in making an intelligent, educated decision; that is in ensuring patient autonomy.

As nurses we should not be regarded as a threat by our medical colleagues, but rather recognised as a source of support and information that has yet to be harnessed to improve the overall care for the patient.

References
Ashworth, P. (1984) Accounting for ethics. *Nursing Mirror*, **158**, 10, 34-6.
Barkes, P. (1979) Bioethics and informed consent in American health care delivery. *Journal of Advanced Nursing*, **4**, 23-38.
Besch, L. (1979) Informed consent: A patient's right. *Nursing Outlook*, January, 32-35.
Bucklin, R. (1975) Informed consent: past present and future. *Legal Medical Annual*, 203-214.
Ferguson, V. (1981) Informed consent: given the facts. *Nursing Mirror*, **155**, 35.
Goldie, L. (1982) The ethics of telling the patient. *Journal of Medical Ethics*, 8, 128-133.

Hanks, G. (1983) Management of symptoms in advanced cancer. *Postgraduate Update,* 1691-1702.

Hayward, J. (1973) Information – a prescription against pain. RCN, London.

Kennedy, I. (1980) Medical ethics are not separate from but part of other ethics. Reith Lecture, *The Listener,* 27 November.

MacDonald, M. and Mever, K. (1976) Medicolegal notes: informed consent. *The Mount Sinai Journal of Medicine,* **43,** 104-107.

Marks, M. A Patient's guide to Chemotherapy – Your Questions Answered. Royal Marsden Hospital Patient Guide series.

Martin, A.J. (1977) Consent to treatment. *Nursing Times,* **73,** 810-11.

Meisel, A. (1975) Informed consent – the rebuttal. *Journal of American Medical Association,* **234,** 6, 615.

Miller, L. (1980) Informed Consent. *Journal of American Medical Association,* **24,** 2661-2662.

Wells, R. (1979) Who, what and when to tell. *Nursing Mirror,* **75,** 22-3.

25

Exploring nurses' attitudes to Aids

Philip Burnard, MSc, RGN, RMN, DipN, Cert Ed, RNT
Lecturer in Nursing Studies, University of Wales College of Medicine, Cardiff

As research continues for answers to the Aids problem, society finds various ways to cope with the disease, prevent its spread and to cope with the emotions it arouses. It seems clear from media coverage that many people react to Aids with fear and prejudice, which can lead to irrational fears about the disease and a temptation to ostracise various groups of people in society, most notably perhaps, gay men. This situation may be partially remedied if people explore their fears and doubts, and in the process develop further self-awareness and empathy. It is particularly important that nurses, who are often in the front line of treatment and care, identify some of their attitudes and feelings towards the issues raised by Aids. If they do not, they risk their unidentified attitudes 'leaking' through their professional presentation of self. It is tempting to believe that we can easily hide our real feelings, but in fact they are usually conveyed in subtle, often non-verbal ways, and are as clear to others as if we had spelled them out.

A self-awareness workshop

This chapter identifies some methods of exploring such attitudes and feelings. The exercises described grew out of a counselling and self-awareness workshop for Aids counsellors and may be modified for use by a variety of nursing groups. They can also be used to develop general counselling and interpersonal skills. The workshop outlined here may best suit a group of 12–15 nurses, but it can be modified for use by larger groups. It is useful if the group sits in a circle and if the leader of the group has some experience of group facilitation. There is a considerable amount of literature on small group facilitation, and many nurse tutors are now developing the specific skills involved in organising and running small learning groups.

The first stage in the workshop involves introductions. A simply way of ensuring each person in the group knows the others is to invite members to pair off and talk to their partner for five minutes. During that time it is suggested that each person finds out five things about their partner (including, of course, her or his name!). The group members then reconvene in the larger group and each person in turn introduces their partner to the group. This process should be taken slowly, as it is part of the workshop that Knowles (1975) describes as 'climate setting'. Group members are coming to terms with each other and getting over some of their initial shyness – not that this will necessarily be true of every member. Some people find group activities particularly difficult and this should be respected throughout the day: no-one should feel under pressure to take part in any activity that they do not freely choose to participate in.

After these initial introductions, it is helpful if two slow 'name rounds' are undertaken. Each person in turn articulates the name by which they wish to be known throughout the workshop. The accent should be on 'slow', here – if the rounds are rushed, names are soon forgotten. The slow pace of the round helps further in allowing people to settle down and feel comfortable in the group. With help from the facilitator, the second 'round' can usually be slower than the first! After these two rounds, group members may be invited to ask the names of any group members they still do not remember.

Icebreaking

If group members already know each other, one or two 'icebreaker' activities may be used to begin the workshop. For example: participants stand up and wander around the room. At a signal from the facilitator, they stop and spend a few minutes sharing something with the person nearest them, then wander around again until the facilitator signals again for them to stop and talk to another person for a few moments. This can be repeated a number of times until the atmosphere in the room feels friendly and relaxed. Suitable topics for sharing in this activity include:

● interests away from work;

● holidays looked forward to, and

● feelings about being a member of the group.

After introductions, the facilitator outlines the aim of the workshop: to explore personal feelings and attitudes towards Aids. Again, it can be restated that members should feel free only to participate in the exercises that they elect to participate in. 'Ground rules' and domestic issues should be clarified too: the group may wish to have a policy on smoking or non-smoking, and arrangements may have to be agreed upon about breaks, meals or refreshment periods and so forth.

The next stage involves a simple pairs activity to encourage people to talk and listen to each other. The group pairs off, and each member talks to their partner for five minutes while the partner listens. It should be emphasised that this is not a *conversation*, the listener *listens*. Topics that may be suggested for this exercise include the following:

● My strengths and shortcomings as a nurse.

- My strengths and shortcomings as a person.

- How I imagine other people see me.

Other topics may be generated by group members or the facilitator. After the first five minutes, the pairs switch roles and the 'listener' becomes the 'talker'. After a further five minutes, the pairs reform into the larger group and the facilitator invites them to share their reactions to the exercise. A decision may be made by the facilitator and the group as to whether or not the group will share the *content* of the exercise – what was talked about in the pairs.

This activity helps further develop group cohesion, and when the content of the exercise is shared, it is usual for people to realise how much they have in common. Carl Rogers (1967) noted this when he said "what is most personal is most general". In other words, what I worry about is probably what you worry about, and vice versa.

Reactions to Aids

The pairs format can be continued as the workshop moves on to explore attitudes and feelings about Aids. Group members pair off again, and each 'talker' considers aloud her or his reaction to the question "how would I feel and what would I do if I discovered that I or a member of my family had Aids?" The talkers verbalise their thoughts to the 'listeners', who, again, do not comment but only listen. After five minutes, roles are reversed and the listeners consider and verbalise answers to the question, to their partners. The facilitator asks the listeners to note their reaction to what they hear. Sometimes the process of hearing another person express personal issues triggers off all sorts of hidden feelings in the listener. Such feelings, when they surface, can do much to help listeners to clarify their *own* thoughts and feelings.

After the second five minute period, the group reconvenes and the facilitator invokes a discussion of the activity – a 'catalytic' approach is useful (Heron, 1986). This involves the facilitator only using interventions that encourage people to say more:

- open questions;
- reflections of thought and feeling;
- clarifying statements.

This is not the time for information giving or 'teaching' in the traditional sense. The process is of sharing information, feelings and reactions, and new learning arises out of this sharing of personal information (Kolb, 1984). Again, if this discussion is allowed to develop slowly and thoughtfully, the reflective period following the pairs exercise can generate many valuable similarities and differences between group members. The acknowledgement and appreciation of individual differences in this way can enhance self-awareness. It is sometimes surprising and painful to realise that others do not always view the world and the people who live in it as we do! On the other hand, as we noted above, it is surprising how often we share the same anxieties.

It is important that everyone gets a fair hearing and that no one member lionises the discussion. The facilitator should also be prepared to 'rescue' any member who is, for any reason, picked on by another. Certain key themes may emerge from the discussion, and the facilitator may choose to note these down, either on a large flip-chart sheet or on a note pad for the later production of a handout to serve as a memory aid for group members. It is helpful to take a break after this group discussion – often (ironically) it is during these breaks that some of the 'real' talking takes place and group members get to know each other much better.

After the break, the group can go straight into another pairs exercise to consider the question "what do my reactions to Aids tell me about myself?" The same format is followed as for the previous exercise. Both partners consider and verbalise answers to the question for five minutes, then the larger group reconvenes to process the activity as outlined above. Again, the facilitator may choose to note down frequent reactions as a memory aid. If the key issues are written on a large flip-chart sheet, this can be fixed to the wall and serve as a constant aide memoire throughout the rest of the day.

After this third pairs activity and group discussion, the group is then invited to form into smaller groups of about five or six people. These groups then carry out the following exercise in parallel. These concurrent group exercises may be followed through in the same room or the groups may move out of the room for increased privacy.

The hot seat

Each member of the small group takes five minutes to occupy what is called the 'hotseat'. While there, that person may be asked questions by any other members of the group (and by the facilitator) on any subject. If they find the question too difficult or prefer not to answer, they may merely say 'pass' and the questioning moves on. On no account should anyone feel forced to answer questions, and those asking are asked to reflect on why they chose those particular questions. After one person has occupied the hotseat for five minutes, she or he nominates another member of the group to occupy the seat and the cycle is repeated until each member of the group (including the facilitator) has had a turn.

This exercise is particularly useful for extending group members' self-awareness through sharing personal information and clarifying ideas in a small group session. The previous pairs exercise called for self-disclosure directed by the individual, while this calls for self-disclosure through other people's direction. This creates a useful balance and the small group work helps to further group cohesion. Following the small group work, the larger group reconvenes and a free discussion follows.

By this stage, an open and comfortable atmosphere will normally have developed and it is in this period that the other issues relating to feelings about Aids may be pursued. Other questions that may be discussed here include the following:

- What does the discussion, so far, tell me about myself?
- How do I feel about my own sexuality?
- What are the implications of all this for me, as a nurse?
- Do I know enough about Aids?
- What do I tell my children about Aids?

My 10 year-old daughter has just read the last question, over my shoulder as I wrote it and confronted me with the question "well, what *do* you tell your children about Aids?". Such questions always seem easier to discuss in adult groups!

After the group discussion, there is often a request for factual information about Aids, and this should be available either in the form of printed matter (available from a variety of sources, including the RCN and the Terrence Higgins Trust) or as a short theory input from the facilitator. In a sense, this second option is the less appropriate, given the nature of the workshop. A theory input at this stage can cause the workshop to develop rather suddenly into a traditional teaching session and its open and disclosing atmosphere may be lost. If there is considerable demand for a more formal theory input it is sometimes possible to arrange such a session at a later date. It is notable, however, that a number of Aids counsellors (as opposed to nurses-as-Aids counsellors) consider themselves well informed about the 'factual' side of the Aids issue but are less well prepared to face the emotional issues at stake. Such issues may usefully be explored in a workshop like this.

Videos

If there is time, video films can be used at this stage to encourage further discussion and consolidation of learning. A useful technique is to use short episodes of videos as triggers for discussion. Alternatively, home-made trigger videos may be prepared by the facilitator, illustrating particular and controversial aspects of the Aids problem. It is useful if such pre-prepared short videos relate specifically to nursing. The use of video in this way is often better than showing a whole film, because the group remains intact and the cohesiveness developed during the day is not lost through lengthy concentration on another focus. Subject matter for such film clips may include:

- counselling homosexual partners;
- helping people cope with bereavement;
- breaking bad news.

The workshop closes with group members sharing in the large group their thoughts about the day. This may be done formally by the use of two rounds:

1. "what I have liked least about the day", and
2. "what I have liked most about the day".

This can be done informally by group members verbalising what they have learned from the day. The choice of which type of evaluation will lie with the facilitator who must judge the atmosphere and the appropriateness of either approach.

It is important for nurses to clarify their feelings about Aids. They will increasingly be looked to for information about the disease and many will find themselves nursing people with Aids. It is tempting to think that feelings about Aids, people with Aids and nursing Aids patients is a 'personal' affair, but Aids is too big and too difficult an issue for that to be an appropriate response. It is everyone's concern.

The workshop outlined here offers one approach to exploring feelings, values and attitudes related to the disease. It may be followed up by further workshops on counselling skills for nurses who have responsibility in this field. It is important that Aids counselling is much more than 'information giving' and all nurses who work as Aids counsellors will need thorough preparation in developing effective and caring counselling skills.

Bibliography
Altman, D. (1986) Aids and the New Puritanism. Pluto Press, London.
    A challenging book about the Aids crisis.
Burnard, P. and Chapman, C. M. (1988) Professional and Ethical Issues in Nursing. Wiley, Chichester.
    A useful source of ideas about ethical issues in nursing.
Daniels, V.G. (1986) Aids – Questions and Answers. Cambridge Medical Books, London.
    A practical, readable guide to aids-related issues.
Health Education Council (1986) Aids – What Everyone Needs to Know. HEC, London.
    More easy-to-read information.
Richardson, D. (1987) Women and the Aids Crisis. Pandora Press, London.
    A vital book for anyone concerned with Aids.
Royal College of Nursing (1986) Nursing Guidelines on the Management of Patients in Hospital and the Community Suffering From Aids. RCN, London.
    Useful information about nursing care.

References
Heron, J. (1986) Six Category Intervention Analysis (2nd Edition). Human Potential Research Project, University of Surrey, Guildford.
Kolb, D. (1984) Experimental Learning. Prentice Hall, Englewood Cliffs, New Jersey.
Knowles, M. (1975) Self-Directed Learning. Cambridge Books, New York.
Rogers, C.R. (1967) On Becoming a Person. Constable, London.

26

Do we discriminate against Aids patients?

Ian Peate, RGN

Nurse Teacher, Continuing Education Department, Barnet Health Authority

The researcher's own experience has shown that a bias exists among nurses against Aids sufferers, or patients suspected of being human immunodeficiency virus (HIV) antibody positive. Working in an A & E unit I found whenever an effeminate male, or even a male patient who gave his next of kin as another male came into the department, he was immediately classed as a potential Aids sufferer. Upon this classification he had to have his blood pressure taken by the junior nurse, who was told to wear two pairs of surgical gloves to do this. The purpose of this study is to examine nurses' views of patients suffering from the acquired immune deficiency syndrome (Aids).

Unpopular patients

Stockwell (1972) attempted to determine whether there were some patients the caring team enjoyed caring for more than others. She also examined the reasons why, and whether there was a measurable difference in the nursing care afforded to the most and least popular patients. Stockwell goes on to state the reasons for patient unpopularity. These included factors related to personality and physical defects such as deafness. Foreign patients and those who stayed in hospital longer than three months proved to be more significantly unpopular than others.

Neuberger (1986) states that the lack of compassion in dealing with Aids victims (sic) is sad and depressing. She cites the case of a woman, married to an HIV positive haemophilliac, who was to undergo major surgery. The woman was warned that staff may find it difficult to treat her kindly, and was asked to be "as supportive as possible". One wonders why the patient, facing major surgery should be expected to give support to her carers, rather than receive it from them. Neuberger suggests part of the reason is undoubtedly a misconceived notion that people with Aids have contracted the disease through their own fault. It is the expression of prejudice against male homosexuals and drug abusers, ignoring haemophilliacs, children and spouses.

Hadden (1986) describes the first time she cared for an Aids sufferer. She speaks of the feelings of insecurity and says she found less time to talk to that patient for some reason. It was not until she spoke to the patient's family and identified him as an individual that she began to see him as a man rather than a disease. Hadden ends her article by saying she began to see Aids patients not as a threat, but as sufferers, struggling to survive. They, like other patients need the care that nurses can and should provide.

A letter written by Napier (1985) a lecturer in postgraduate nursing studies, states quite frankly that he has no sympathy with homosexuals who contract the disease through performing unnatural sexual acts. He goes on to say the disease is "self-inflicted" and need not have arisen in the first place. Napier continues to make value ridden comments throughout his letter and finishes by saying that what makes Aids more horrific is that a stranger's perverse sexual actions can harm totally unknown 'innocents'.

Examining the problem

Due to the above anecdotal and scientific evidence, I felt it necessary to examine the problem using a scientific approach. It is hoped the results of this study will have implications for the nursing care given to people who are HIV positive or suffering from Aids.

The problem was examined using a modified questionnaire described by Wattley and Müller (1984). They used the study to investigate how a group of nurses studying for the diploma in nursing would assess certain characteristics of two patients, based on a brief description. The description included the patients' age, marital status, occupation, political bias, type of housing, hobbies and medical diagnosis. The patients used in the study were one suffering from cirrhosis of the liver, one with a hernia. The study found a bias towards seeing the hernia patient as having more positive characteristics. This bias emerged after only a brief description of the two patients.

Thus it was decided to present nurses with profiles of two ficticious patients (one with a hernia and one with Aids, but otherwise identical), and ask them to judge them on certain characteristics. It was expected that the Aids patient would be judged more negatively than the hernia patient.

Patient portrait (i)
Is 30 years old.
Married with two children.
Served in the forces.
Votes Labour.
Owns a semi-detached house.
Keen on sport.
Occupation: Technician.
Reason for hospitalisation:- Hernia repair.

Patient portrait (ii)
Is 30 years old.
Married with two children.
Served in the forces.
Votes Labour.
Owns a semi-detached house.
Keen on sport.
Occupation: Technician.
Reason for hospitalisation:- Acquired immune deficiency syndrome (Aids).

Consider the patient characteristics listed below and using a four point scale rate the extent to which you think each will apply to the person described. For example if you think that the patient will be very cheerful then mark him 4, somewhat cheerful 3, somewhat unhappy 2, or very unhappy 1.

1. Cheerful .... Unhappy

2. Pleasant .... Unpleasant

3. Helpful .... Unhelpful

4. Grateful .... Ungrateful

5. Cooperative .... Uncooperative

6. Sense of humour .... Humourless

7. Easy to talk to .... Difficult to talk to

8. Understanding .... Lack of understanding

9. Willing to accept treatment .... Unwilling to accept treatment

10. Keen to get better .... Indifferent

11. Optimistic .... Pessimistic

12. Interesting to nurse .... Uninteresting to nurse

13. Needs a lot of nursing .... Doesn't need a lot of nursing

14. Will make good progress .... Unlikely to progress

15. Ill .... Not very ill

4.. 3.. 2..1

Table 1. The questionnaire.

Methodology

The subjects were 27 randomly selected nurses (a crude selection was made by picking ward names blindly from a hat), two were male and 25 female, comprising 16 RGNs, 10 EN(G)s and one RMN. The study was carried out in a London teaching hospital in October 1986. The total population from which a sample of 30 was drawn was 372 qualified nurses in an acute area working day duty. Originally 30 nurses were approached, but three felt unable to judge the patients' characteristics because they felt they would need to meet the patients before passing any form of judgement on them.

The research tool used was a structured questionnaire (Table 1), the characteristics of which are of a modified form of that used by Stockwell (1972) in her study. The nurses were asked to read about one of the patients (see profiles) who they should imagine was to be admitted to their ward. They were then asked to assess the patient characteristics shown (Table 1). The marking system that was used was a modified Likert four point scale.

Thirteen randomly selected nurses were asked to judge the characteristics of a patient suffering from Aids and 14 judged those of the hernia patient. After these had been assessed the nurses were asked to answer two questions regarding blame and avoidance of the disease on their patient profile.

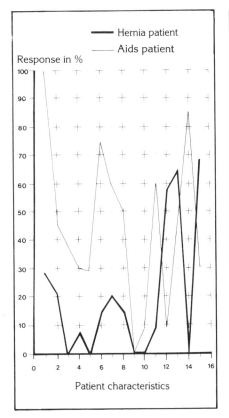

Figure 1. Negative responses for both hernia and Aids patients, represented in percentages.

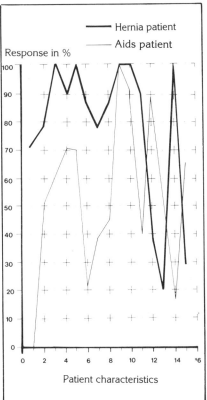

Figure 2. Positive responses for both hernia and Aids patients, represented in percentages.

Results of the study

To analyse the two sets of results concerning the patients' characteristics, the grades on the scale were combined such that all those marked three or four (the positive end of the scale) for a particular characteristic were counted together, as were those marked either one or two (the negative end of the scale). The results are shown in percentages in Figures 1 and 2, thus, for the characteristic number one, cheerful–unhappy the patient suffering with Aids was scored three or four by no nurses and one or two by 13. The same characteristic for the hernia patient was awarded three or four by 10 nurses and one or two by four nurses. This combination of scores makes it easier to make the comparisons between data for the two groups.

The set questions were:

1. To what extent do you think the patient can be held responsible for the disorder?

2. To what extent do you think the patient could have avoided the disorder?

In response to the first question regarding the Aids patient, 46 per cent felt he was somewhat to blame, 46 per cent felt he was a little to blame and 8 per cent felt he was not at all to blame. For the same question regarding the hernia patient, 22 per cent felt he was somewhat to blame, 50 per cent that he was a little to blame and 28 per cent that he was not at all to blame.

In response to the second question, 70 per cent felt the Aids patient could have avoided the disorder somewhat and 30 per cent that he could have done a little to avoid it. For the hernia patient the responses were 22 per cent that he could have avoided it somewhat and 78 per cent that he could have avoided it a little.

Apportioning blame

The two patient profiles used in this study vary in only one characteristic, that of the patient's disease. One group of subjects assessed a man with a hernia, while the other assessed a man with Aids, an illness that may, by some, be associated with a lifestyle that is different, or alternative. In such cases it is probably easier to attribute blame to the patient for having 'acquired the disease'.

The results show that these subjects judged the Aids patient more negatively than the hernia patient on many characteristics.

It was judged that the patient suffering from Aids would be less helpful, less grateful, less cooperative, have less of a sense of humour and be more difficult to talk to than the 'same' patient suffering from a hernia. While the hernia patient is said to have a good prognosis, the Aids patient is not.

Some tentative conclusions can be made concerning how nurses may perceive two different types of patient. The study has demonstrated that nurses are capable of judging patients differently simply on the patient's medical diagnosis. Stockwell's study (1972) demonstrated that the least popular patients receive a lower standard of care than the more popular patients.

Miller (1979) concludes that to understand nurses' attitudes towards their patients, one must take into account the nurse's individual factors – her social background and values. The nurse's personality may also be related to the type of organisational structure she belongs to although this is debatable. Ryland and King (1982) have indicated that a patient who has overdosed and is admitted to a hospital's A & E unit is likely to be less popular than the patient admitted to the same unit with an acute attack of bronchitis, despite the fact that the bronchitis may have been exacerbated by the patient overdosing himself with cigarettes. We might then expect that the patient suffering from Aids would be similarly unpopular. Such a fact would have important implications for nusing care. Patient care will not be as effective as it could be if nurses have negative feelings about the people to whom they deliver care. These feelings could seriously damage the patient's health further.

Education

It is felt that there should be better education for nurses with regard to the care of Aids patients, covering such subjects as the immune system, the aetiology of the syndrome, and the needs of the person with Aids or those who are HIV positive. This could come in the form of continuing education or as a post basic course. Learner nurses should be educated on the subject early in their nurse education, support groups for nurses who are finding it difficult to cope with caring for people with Aids should be made available. Only when nurses are aware of their fears, biases and prejudices will they be able to give the care that the person with Aids, or any other person, deserves and has a right to. It would appear that there is a need for more studies to be carried out in this area in order to identify further the implications for nursing care.

Although this study was not as big as Stockwell's nor was it carried out using real patients, the results are similar. They demonstrate that as professionals, we too have certain biases in the way we judge and view people. The study points to the need for nurses to be aware of their own biases in predicting behaviour and for them to counteract this when caring for certain types of patients.

It must be understood that it is not only members of the homosexual community who have contracted the disease, there are other members of our society who are at risk and may fall foul of the disease, and also that homosexuals with Aids should not be blamed for their condition.

Acknowledgements
I would like to express my gratitude to all of the many fine people who made it possible for me to carry out this study. I am indebted to the nursing staff on the wards in which the study was carried out. Special thanks go to Miss Janet E. Pearson who became my mentor, statistician and friend.

References
Hadden, L. (1986) My first Aids patient. *RN*, March, 51.
Miller, A.E. (1979) Nurses' attitudes towards their patients. *Nursing Times*, **75**, 1929-1932.
Napier, B. (1985) Letter. *Nursing Mirror*, **161**, 18, 11.
Neuberger, J. (1986) Fear and loathing. *Nursing Mirror*, **82**, 22.
Ryland R. and King, (1982). An overdose of attitudes. *Nursing Mirror*, **23**, 154, 40-41.
Stockwell, F. (1972) The Unpopular Patient. Royal College of Nursing, London.
Wattley, L.A. and Muller, D.J. (1984) Investigating Psychology: A Practical Approach for Nursing. Harper and Row, London.

Bibliography
Anderson, D. (1986) AIDS; an update on what we know now. *RN*, March, 54-56.
  A good general update.

Coleman, D.A. (1986) How To Care For AIDS Patients. *RN*, July, 17-21.
 A comprehensive look at nursing care of people with AIDS.
Cook, M. (1979) Perceiving Others, The Psychology of Interpersonal Perception. Methuen, London.
 A look at what affects our perception of people.
Darling, V.H. and Rogers, J. (1986) Nursing; Research For Practising Nurses. MacMillan, London.
 A guide to understanding research.
Sheehan, J. (1985) Starting the study. *Nursing Mirror,* **160,** 17-18.
Sheehan, J. (1985) Reviewing the literature. *Nursing Mirror,* **160,** 29-30.
Sheehan, J. (1985) Selecting the right method. *Nursing Mirror,* **160,** 19-20.
Sheehan, J. (1985) Collecting the data. *Nursing Mirror,* **160,** 25-26.
Sheehan, J. (1985) Presenting the results. *Nursing Mirror,* **160,** 36-37.
 This series is a good step by step guide to research.

27

The spiritual needs of atheists and agnostics

Philip Burnard, MSc, RGN, RMN, DipN, Cert Ed, RNT.
Lecturer in Nursing Studies, University of Wales College of Medicine, Cardiff.

There is, currently in nursing a realisation of the importance of the patient's spiritual needs. However, these needs are frequently couched in terms of religion or religious belief (Sampson, 1982). This chapter examines the notion of the spiritual needs of the atheist or agnostic.

What is spiritual need?

First we may consider what is meant by the term 'spiritual need'. It is perhaps best understood in terms of a search for meaning (Frankl, 1963; Burnard, 1986, 1987). It would appear that most of us need to make sense of our lives in terms of some sort of meaning, but while some invest that meaning through a religious framework, others do not. The 'believers'; however, seem to be better catered for than the 'unbelievers'. Indeed, most admission procedures involve, at some stage, a question regarding religion. Many unbelievers, nervous of expressing such a position, may find it more comfortable to have themselves marked down as 'Church of England' or other religion. It may be time for us to consider other ways of posing questions about spirituality.

Of course the world cannot be divided only into 'believers' and 'unbelievers'. Many people give little thought to spiritual issues or find little relevance in them. To adopt the position of atheist or agnostic is to have considered the issue and to have made a conscious decision.

The denial of a God

What, then, *are* atheism and agnosticism? Atheism is the unequivocal denial of the possible existence of God. The atheist is the 'unbeliever'. It is interesting for us to ponder our reaction to such a position. Do we respond by seeing such people as 'wrong'? Or believe they need only to reflect further for clarification? Do they need more education to bring them to the truth; or do we accept them as they are? Various reactions are possible; the least acceptable seems to be the notion that somehow the unbeliever is 'wrong' and the believer 'right'. Belief in God involves a 'leap of faith' (Kierkegaard, 1959). There can be no ultimate proof of the existence or non-existence of God. We either believe or do not.

Neither does the position of unbelief necessarily preclude any sort of moral position. An unbeliever is quite as able to lead a moral life as a believer. Indeed, Simone de Beauvoir argued that the unbeliever had to lead a *more* moral life than the believer, because, having no final arbiter for right and wrong, the unbeliever is necessarily thrown back onto his or her own decision making as a guide to conduct. Believers can be 'forgiven'; the unbelievers must forgive themselves.

Atheists usually have to look beyond the concept of God for meaning. This does not mean they do not have spiritual needs; in terms of a search for meaning, they are just as vital as for the believer. Some atheists will find meaning through their work or their relationships, others may find a sense of meaning in secular humanism. Secular humanism should not be confused with 'humanistic psychology' (Shaffer, 1978). Humanistic psychology is a branch of psychology centring on individual human experience. Secular humanism is a particular set of beliefs about the world without a notion of God.

The basic argument of secular humanism is perhaps best outlined by Blackham (1968). Briefly the argument is that people are alone in that there is no God. Because they are alone, they are responsible for themselves. They also have the joint responsibility of being responsible for all other people. In acting for themselves, they should act as though they were acting for all mankind. To do less than this is selfishness and not, according to Blackham, secular humanism. Such a philosophy offers an immediate sense of meaning: we are responsible for ourselves and for others. As a result, the 'golden rule' applies: we should treat others as we ourselves would wish to be treated. This, then, is the basis for morality and meaning without recourse to belief in God.

Again, however, it should be noted that it is possible to be an atheist without necessarily accepting the premises outlined by secular humanists. Some people choose not to believe in God and do not find it necessary to find an 'alternative' set of principles by which to make sense of their lives.

Neither believer or unbeliever

Agnostics, on the other hand, are in a slightly different position. They argue that because it is impossible to prove or disprove the existence of God, silence on the issue is the only wise position (Bullock and Stallybrass, 1977). They are neither believer nor unbeliever but hold that discussion on the matter is necessarily misplaced because, in the end, such an issue can only ever be a matter of faith. Again, such a position does not, of itself, rule out the need for meaning or morality. Agnostics, like atheists, still need to discover or invest meaning in what they do or how they live. Some may argue that the only meaning that *can* be found in life is that which we as individuals invest in it ourselves (Kopp, 1972). In other words, there is no ultimate meaning for the way things are; *we* as people bring meaning to what we do.

Another, more popular use of the term 'agnostic' is where it describes the person who is undecided about the existence or otherwise of God. Clearly many people will also fall into this category.

These are two thumbnail sketches of two positions alternative to that of belief in God. It is argued here that such positions are just as valid as those adopted by people who claim to be believers.

The nursing role

There are many situations in which such positions need to be considered in nursing. One of the questions usually asked on a patient's admission may relate to that person's 'religion'. Such a question leaves no doubt that the accepted position is that of 'believer'. We need to think long and hard about how we may pose questions about belief or unbelief without making such questions *leading* questions.

We also need to consider the sorts of value-judgements we may make about other people's belief systems. If we are believers, do we judge, harshly, the unbeliever? If, on the other hand, we are unbelievers, do we dismiss the believer? It is important that we acknowledge that *our* belief system may not coincide with that of our patient, and that we do not prosyletise or evangelise for *either* position. As nurses, we are not required (while we are at work) to convert others to belief or unbelief.

There are other more delicate questions. Can we accept, for instance, that the unbeliever may not see the need for the conventional funeral service? 'Secular' forms of service are available through national secular societies. Can we acknowledge, also, that death need not be fearful for the unbeliever? Nor need it be fearful for unbelieving relatives.

The whole question of belief systems and value systems seems to underlie the way we approach the issue of patients' spiritual needs. Nurses need first to clarify *their own* belief and value systems before they can help patients with such 'ultimate' questions. Value clarification exercises may be useful here (Simon, Howe and Kirschenbaum, 1978).

It would do a great disservice to a wide variety of ways of addressing spiritual matters if the term 'spiritual' was only connoted as being to do with religious matters. Nurses need to be open minded in their approach to this vital aspect of nursing care.

References

Blackham, H.J. (1986) Humanism, Pelican, Harmondsworth.
Bullock, A. and Stallybrass, O. (eds) (1977) The Fontana Dictionary of Modern Thought. Fontana, London.
Burnard, P. (1987) Spiritual distress and the nursing response; theoretical considerations and counselling skills. *Journal of Advanced Nursing;* **12,** 377-382.
Frankl, V. (1963) Man's Search for Meaning. Washington Square Books, New York.
Kierkegaard, S. (1959) Either/Or: Vol 1. Doubleday, New York.
Kopp, S. (1974) If You Meet the Buddha on the Road, Kill Him! Sheldon Press, London.
Samson, C. (1982) The Neglected Ethic: Religious and Cultural Factors in the Care of Patients. McGraw Hill, Maidenhead, Berkshire.
Shaffer, J.P.B. (1978) Humanistic Psychology. Prentice Hall, Englewood Cliffs, New Jersey.
Simon, S.B., Howe, L.W. and Kirschenbaum, H. (1978) Values Clarification: Revised Edition. A and W Visual Library, New York.

28

Why do adolescents smoke?

Alison Stewart, RGN, RM, BSc, MSc,
Staff Midwife, Bristol Maternity Hospital

Judy Orme, BSc,
Research Assistant, International Centre for Child Studies

Smoking is a controversial subject, at times arousing emotions and reactions similar to those engendered by politics and religion. Even with the proven associated health hazards people continue to smoke. In 1986 35 per cent of men and 31 per cent of women smoked in the UK (OPCS Monitor, 1988). While smokers are now a minority of the population, the habit is still a major preventable cause of premature death. As a result, with regard to health issues the habit maintains a high profile in the public awareness. Action against smoking has been two-fold: helping existing smokers to stop (Kendall, 1986), and preventing the habit becoming established. Preventive education means focusing on children, and realising smoking in childhood and adolescence is widespread.

Adolescent smoking

A national survey of smoking, conducted by the Office of Population Census and Surveys (OPCS), among secondary school children in England and Wales in 1988, revealed that 10 per cent smoked regularly (>1 cigarette per week) compared with 13 per cent in 1984. More than half claimed to have never smoked (Goddard, 1988). This apparent downward trend is encouraging, but the information that one in 10 children smokes regularly indicates the potential health risks accruing in this generation. It is estimated that 40 times more young men who are regular smokers will die as a consequence of smoking than will die in road traffic accidents (Peto, 1980). Recognising the problem entails devising some action to try and reduce this hazard as far as possible, for example formulating anti-smoking material. The aim must ultimately be to try and ensure that children neither 'drift' into smoking, nor are coerced into it: at best it should be an informed choice.

Models of smoking

Exponents from various disciplines have tried to create models to explain why people smoke. These have had psychological, psychosocial, pharmacological and genetic bases. However, it remains difficult to incorporate the different elements into a comprehensive model which will apply to all individuals. The work of developmental theorists is of considerable use in trying to understand this behaviour. Smoking is then seen as a process with different stages such as preparation, initiation, establishment and maintenance.

Who is smoking?

The 1988 OPCS survey reported that of secondary school children, 11 per cent of girls and eight per cent of boys were smoking regularly; while more boys had tried it and then not pursued the habit. However, boys smoke more cigarettes than girls. Similar proportions of both sexes had given up smoking (10 per cent); slightly more boys (57 per cent) than girls 53 per cent) had never smoked. The sex differentiated smoking behaviour suggests different factors are involved in the decision to smoke. Girls may be more conscious of using cigarettes to try and regulate their weight or to emulate a 'cool', sexually attractive woman. Boys may be more concerned with limitations smoking may place on athletic prowess.

Among 11-16 year-olds, as age increases, the proportion of never-smokers decreases, with regular smoking being most prevalent in the older age groups of 14-16 years. In the Brigantia survey (Charlton, 1984a) of 16,000 nine to 19-year-olds of those having tried a cigarette, one per cent claimed to have had a puff of a cigarette by the age of four.

Family   Much childhood social learning occurs in the home as children copy other members of the family. In the Brigantia survey, children were twice as likely to be smokers if their parents smoked.

Peers   Other studies have concentrated on the effects of peer group pressure. Bewley and Bland (1977) in a study of 491 schoolchildren aged 10-10½ found that 76 per cent of smokers had friends who smoked compared to 36 per cent of non-smokers. Inevitably, friends can exert considerable influence and act as or sources of supply.

School   The milieu provided at school with curriculum teaching, teacher/pupil example and relations of different peer groups, can act as a stimulus or a deterrent on becoming a smoker. Varying rates of smoking can occur between different types of school in the same geographical area (Banks et al, 1978). In view of the instability of many home situations, schools may be a major influence, representing a constant feature in a changing childhood. Nash (1987) reported that 14-16 year-olds appeared to smoke partly for the pleasure of rebelling against school authority. Bewley and Bland (1977) found that both children's self-ratings and those of teachers assessed non-smokers as academically better than smokers. This may be due to time taken smoking – or obtaining income for it – having a detrimental effect on school performance or due to low-achievers boosting their morale by smoking.

Adolescence is commonly associated with a period of crisis and confusion as the individual changes from a child to an adult. The dissonance our society creates in terms of employment prospects, Youth Training Schemes, sexual freedom and so on heightens teenagers' sense of their anomalous position. Self-esteem and confidence may be low, and smoking may raise morale and reduce tension.

As a smoker

Each adolescent's perception of the effects of smoking will depend on how smoking is learned to be associated with changes in physical/mental states. These changes can then be labelled as pleasant or aversive and the example of family and friends can contribute to this.

With regard to future smoking behaviour some adolescents in the OPCS survey who were not currently smoking anticipated that they would smoke before leaving school. Grouped by current smoking status this included never-smokers (4 per cent), tried smoking once (10 per cent) and used to smoke (29 per cent). The fact that far fewer in these groups thought that they would become regular smokers after leaving school suggests the importance of tobacco usage in school-culture; a function which may change when leaving school. As might be expected regular smokers were more likely to anticipate continuing smoking beyond school-years (63 per cent). Adolescence is a time in which young people try out different roles, images and behaviours. The danger occurs when adolescents find it difficult to give up an established habit.

Health

The detrimental consequences of smoking on health are well documented and effects may occur very early in a smoker's life. In children aged 10-12½ years, respiratory symptoms (eg coughs) correlated with smoking. Regular smokers reported more symptoms than occasional smokers, who reported more than never-smokers (Bewley and Bland, 1976). Future mortality and morbidity effects appear to be increased when smoking starts before the age of 15 years (Hammond, 1966). Of particular current concern are the potential health risks of girls smoking, and also using the contraceptive pill.

Leisure

Banks et al (1978), found smokers were more likely to go to a youth club, go round with a group of their own age and have a friend of the opposite sex, rather than stay at home reading. Obviously, activities create opportunities to experiment and to conform to the existing peer culture.

Media and advertising

Television advertising of cigarettes was banned in 1965, but tobacco companies now use subtle pressures such as sports sponsorship to obtain viewing time exposure to brand names. Films and soap-operas can provide both negative and positive images of smoking through heroes and anti-heroes, which may exert a counter pressure to attempts to inform children of the risks of smoking. The tobacco industry tries to justify poster advertising by claiming they may increase brand awareness and encourage smokers to change to lower tar cigarettes. However, it has been argued that the advertisements contain minimal information and may also influence non-smokers (Chapman, 1985).

Beliefs about smoking

Knowledge about smoking comes from numerous sources, in particular, significant others, such as the family, and may determine children's smoking behaviour. For example, if all the family and friends smoke, smoking may appear a natural activity like eating and sleeping. Charlton (1984b) found that smokers associated 'calms nerves' with smoking, while never-smokers and ex-smokers associated negative aspects of the behaviour such as it being a waste of money and smelly. However, knowledge is not always applied to self. A sample of 16-17 year-olds revealed more regular smokers than non-smokers associated cigarettes with the word 'cancer'. They also exhibited a well developed awareness of the health risks yet continued to smoke (Charlton, 1982). This might suggest that the information of a long-term risk has little impact on short-term decisions to smoke – the risk is not perceived as 'real'.

Health education

The extent to which children are exposed to health education varies between schools. In the OPCS 1986 survey, 42 per cent of secondary school children had received a lesson on smoking in the previous year. (Goddard and Ikin, 1987). By 1988 this had risen to 52 per cent. The percentage was lowest among first-years and highest among fifth-years, so many of the early smokers are not being reached in time. Subjects such as diet and hygiene continue to receive a larger coverage than emotive issues like smoking and alcohol (Goddard, 1988).

The nurse's role

Nurses have a major role in combating adolescent smoking. The aim must be three-fold: discourage individuals starting or continuing; provide realistic, understandable information about the risks, so that those smoking are making an informed choice, and provide sufficient support for those who choose to give up smoking.

In schools   School nurses and health visitors have extended their role beyond routine screening examinations to involvement in the provision of curriculum health education. It is important to ensure that smoking is not neglected in favour of more topical areas such as AIDS or more neutral ones such as diet and hygiene. Since many children try smoking at an early age, discussions about smoking may be appropriate even at early primary school age. It is important to appreciate the diversity of influences for adolescents and children smoking. Formal lectures may be of limited value, since they may not have the scope to confront all the erroneous beliefs which individual smokers may hold such as 'I smoke to be slim', and 'cancer can be cured'. Group discussions using a starting strategy of asking participants what they think/believe about the subject can be invaluable, and are as relevant for non-smokers as smokers. Nurses are likely to find varying opinions and behaviour in different schools, and alternative approaches will be needed to suit particular needs. Ideas for presentations of material include:

• Group discussions on any issue related to smoking. Many programmes in the USA have sought to explore adolescents' self-perceptions and support their self-esteem to enable them to withstand social pressures to conform and smoke.

• Lectures on health risks, physiology of smoking, economic and social aspects of the habit.

• Using the current teaching aids/courses, GCSE has several useful active learning books and there are various TV broadcasts for schools.

• Linking in with national anti-smoking awareness campaigns such as the annual National No-Smoking Day.

Increasing emphasis is being placed on active learner participation and as nurses we need to consider how to use this type of teaching method effectively to communicate our message.

The example of individuals such as teachers and nurses can contribute to the decision to smoke. To discourage children from smoking and then be seen smoking negates the whole message. We need to consider our behaviour and its influence on others in contact with children, eg encouraging schools to adopt a non-smoking policy for staff.

Action in the family   Nurses in any specialty can advise adults about the injurious effects of smoking and the effect parental influence has on children's habits. Future parents may therefore be inculcated with more responsible attitudes towards their children's health.

The primary care team   Nurses working in treatment rooms or offering family planning services can discuss smoking on an individual basis as part of a check-up. In a one-to-one discussion it may be possible to provide specific incentives to an adolescent to give up or not take up smoking. It is particularly important for family planning nurses to try to discover the 'true' smoking habits of teenagers seeking contraception and advise them on the risks of choosing to take the Pill and smoke.

Action in society   This may involve all nurses with measures such as campaigning for the Government to ban all forms of tobacco advertisements and discourage consumption with increased added tax on cigarettes. The problem of smoking at an early age has belatedly received Government attention, with a health campaign to be launched in 1990 directed towards adolescents. Nurses may also be involved in activities with young people such as Guides, Scouts and church clubs, which may provide the opportunity of approaching the subject of smoking in a more social setting than classrooms or surgeries.

Since many adolescents say they intend to stop smoking, there is a need for considerable support and encouragement to help them do so. Many smokers comment that a major problem in giving up is not succumbing to the craving, often when they have apparently successfully stopped. When advising smokers to stop, nurses must consider the feasibility of either setting up counselling/support groups or at least putting the individual in contact with a pre-existing one.

Acknowledgement

To Cancer Research Campaign for funding to undertake the analysis of Youthscan data with reference to smoking. It is hoped that the results from the survey of the third national cohort (16,000 babies born in 1970) at the age of 16 years, will provide information on some of the issues discussed in this chapter.

Useful information

Leaflets and Factsheets produced by ASH 75p for a set of eight factsheets on health aspects and economics of smoking. Margaret Pyke House, 27-35 Mortimer Street, London W1N 7RJ.

Information sheet by GASP, 37 Stokes Croft, Bristol BS1 3PY.

Useful, up-to-date information with some relevance to adolescent issues.

Bibliography

Jacobsen, B. (1986) Beating the Ladykillers. Pluto Press, London.

A broad range of issues including feminist aspects and Third World involvement.

Smoking and Me (1988) HEA, London.

Information about supporting children to resist the pressures to smoke.

References

Banks, M.H. et al (1978) Long-term study of smoking by secondary school children. *Arch. of Dis. in Childhood*, **53**, 12-19.

Bewley, B.R. and Bland, J.M. (1976) smoking and respiratory symptoms in two groups of schoolchildren. *Preventive Medicine*, **5**, 63-69.

Bewley, B.R. and Bland, J.M. (1977) Academic performance and social factors related to cigarette smoking by school children. *British Journal of Preventive and Social Medicine*, **31** 18-24.

Charlton, A. (1984a) The Brigantia smoking survey: a general review. In: Public Education about Cancer. UICC Technical Report Series: 77, 92-102.

Charlton, A. (1984b) Children's opinions about smoking. *Jnl. RCGP*, **34**, 483-87.

Chapman, S. (1985) Cigarette advertising and smoking: a review of the evidence. In: Smoking out the Barons 1986. John Wiley, London.

Goddard, E. (1988) Smoking among secondary schoolchildren in England, 1988. HMSO, London.

Goddard, E. and Ikin, C. (1987) Smoking among secondary schoolchildren in 1986. HMSO, London.

Hammond, E.C. (1966) Smoking in relation to death rates of one million men and women. National Cancer Institute Monograph, 19, 127.

Kendall, S. (1986) Helping people to stop smoking. *The Professional Nurse*, **1**, 120-23.

Nash, J. (1987). Sparking up – smoking and style in school. *Health Ed. Jnl.* **46**, 152-55.

OPCS Monitor Cigarette Smoking: 1972 to 1986, SS 88/1 9/2/88.

Peto, R. (1980) Possible ways of explaining the quantitative dangers of smoking. *Health Ed. Jnl.*, **39**, 2, 45-6.

Index